Solving the SMA Puzzle: Complications of SMN Protein Upregulation

Solving the SMA Puzzle: Complications of SMN Protein Upregulation

heBGG

iUniverse, Inc.
New York Lincoln Shanghai

Solving the SMA Puzzle: Complications of SMN Protein Upregulation

iUniverse books may be ordered through booksellers or by contacting:

iUniverse
2021 Pine Lake Road, Suite 100
Lincoln, NE 68512
www.iuniverse.com
1-800-Authors (1-800-288-4677)

cover art: Amanda Schuermann

ISBN-13: 978-0-595-42833-5 (pbk)
ISBN-13: 978-0-595-87172-8 (ebk)
ISBN-10: 0-595-42833-9 (pbk)
ISBN-10: 0-595-87172-0 (ebk)

Printed in the United States of America

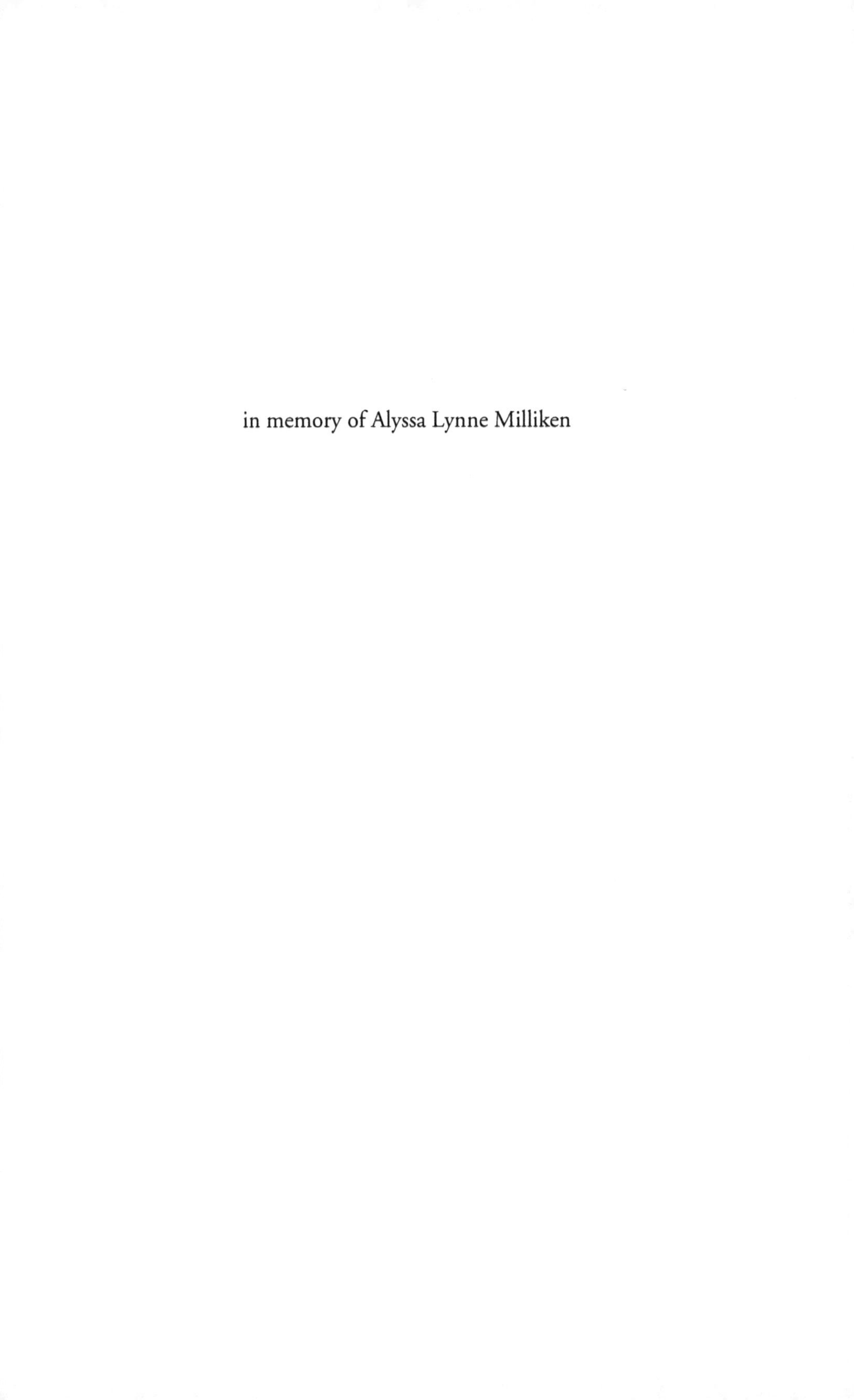

in memory of Alyssa Lynne Milliken

Contents

Author's Note

This essay was originally written as a roadmap for my wife and me to chart our next steps in the search for a cure for our two and one-half year old daughter who has Type I Spinal Muscular Atrophy. Upon completion, it seemed as though the information and research it contains may be of useful benefit for parents who share similar circumstances. However, I need to caution anyone who reads this paper that I am not a doctor, scientist, researcher, or expert in this or any other related field. In writing this paper, I have conducted no experiments to verify my findings.

Rather, I am merely a concerned father and husband who has been profoundly affected by this insidious disease. Ten years ago, my niece Alyssa Milliken died in my twin sister's arms on Christmas Eve at the age of seven months. Now, my own daughter Cassandra suffers from this very disease. A bi-pap ventilator, cough and suction machines, a feeding tube, vigilance and the grace of God keep her with us. Any decisions you make regarding your son or daughter *must* be based on your own research and not my unsubstantiated findings.

My intent in creating this document and making it public is to present an understandable format that describes the very basics of current research and therapy. My intent is to promote further discussion about this disease in hopes of expediting an inevitable cure.

Abstract

This study investigates the extent to which survival of motor neuron protein upregulation is an effective therapy for severe Spinal Muscular Atrophy ("SMA I") patients.

The hypothesis is that if rapid motor neuron death occurs as a result of a lack of survival of motor neuron ("SMN") protein, then post-neuronal death SMN protein upregulation will have a minimally favorable effect (defined as "motor neuron rescue"). The thesis will address the following questions: (1) to what extent and at what point can SMN protein upregulation rescue precious motor neurons, (2) what alternatives exist to SMN protein upregulation, and (3) when SMA I characteristics present, to what extent can motor function be restored?

Using SMA I as its model, this paper researches primary documents including media interviews, newspaper and journal articles, press releases, laboratory reports, meeting minutes, published papers, and personal experience to provide a synthesis for a detailed analysis of the likely outcome of latent SMN protein upregulation on the increasing number of SMA I survivors as well as provide a roadmap of options for those who confront this challenging predicament.

Presently, all three fields of curative therapy (HDAC inhibitors, gene therapy, and stem cell therapy) target SMN protein upregulation. While SMN protein upregulation will undoubtedly have profound curative value for less severe forms of SMA, its effect upon SMA I patients (who develop SMA I at a younger age) remains questionable. For this reason, other methods for motor neuron rescue must be developed without negatively impacting current research.

Although there is no way to assess motor neuron damage without an autopsy, it is generally agreed that early intervention is a vital component to neuronal rescue. In the absence of early intervention, and with a worst-case scenario of ninety percent neuronal death, strategies need to be developed to boost the function of surviving neurons or create a new motor neuron. Although both of these goals are daunting, they are within the realm of possibility.

"I begged the Lord three times to take it away from me.
And He said unto me,
'My grace is sufficient for thee: for my strength is made perfect in weakness.'"

—2 Corinthians 12:8-9

Preface: A Letter to My Wife

Dear Mary,

I am writing this letter after nearly a year of intensive of research. As you know, we are at a point where we are in a position to actively seek a cure for an incurable disease. Of course, this would not be possible without the help of our Lord and Savior Jesus Christ. It is for this reason that I ask you to reflect thus far upon what he has done in our lives since the conception and Easter birth of Cassandra Victoria on April 11, 2004.

Prior to Cassandra, we were chasing the "American" dream, not the one God wanted for us. Neither of us had purpose; we searched for meaning and truth in money, fancy cars, vacations, dinners, and aesthetics. Continued emptiness increased my alcohol and cigarette consumption while you turned to business and the Internet for emotional support and comfort. There was not much meaning to the "dream". In fact, we were separating from each other more and more each day.

Upon the unbelievable realization that we were both carriers of SMA, God began to play a part in our lives even if it was not the way we wanted events to occur. As we drove over the bridge for an Amnio that very day, we succumbed to an overpowering spirit that we should not proceed with the course of doctor recommended actions (amnio and abortion if necessary). Thus, we turned the vehicle around and headed home, into the unknown.

In your womb, we thought Cassandra was much different than Alyssa. We believed that Cassandra was healthy as she kicked quite a bit whereas Alyssa had been prenatally placid. We convinced ourselves that we had dodged a bullet and our personal lives once again took precedence. The horrible thoughts of disaster and doom vanished and our dependence upon God faded ever so faintly to the recesses of our minds.

Cassandra's birth validated our belief that she was indeed healthy. The doctors had confirmed this with her high (9.7) APGAR test. All was well. There was no need to give much more than a few mumbles of thanks to God. Our future was now unfolding just as we had planned; at six months, Cassie would go to daycare, you would resume your new executive position, and I would teach.

Just before her third month, I did not dare mention my growing concern about Cassie's lack of movement in her legs. How could I possibly mention my suspicions to you that the love of our lives could be stricken with the number one genetic killer of babies. However, her three-month check-up revealed nothing unusual. All was well and I was just being over cautious.

What a great weekend! All the terrible thoughts that could not be talked about nor erased from our minds blew away as air from a balloon. We went out to dinner with misplaced relief. We talked about how terrible it would have been; how our lives would have changed, and how we evaded death, bankruptcy from medical bills, and the agonizing pain of loss. No, once again, we believed that fate was not meant for us.

That Monday, reality set in. We needed to take her to Boston to be checked. Her muscle tone didn't look that good after all. There could no longer be any doubt. Cassandra had been stricken with the same disease that mercilessly killed her cousin Alyssa on the eve of Christ's birth seven years earlier.

A wave of despair and despondency barreled into our house. Did you want to live any longer? I know that I did not. I was not strong enough to endure the same wrenching, fiery pain my sister and her family had. I did not want to see my daughter draw her last breath in your arms. I did not want to live without my beautiful daughter. How could I lose the only person that could fill the gaping emptiness of my life? I tried to keep composed driving home from the hospital as you doubled over in convulsing, inconsolable grief. Upon arriving home, I too could no longer bear the pain and despair. I fell to my knees and nearly broke my hands pounding on the hallway floor.

God had been moving. In fact, he had been moving years before we even knew it. Looking back, if I had not gotten that job at Sturgis, events may not have turned out the way they did. I nearly didn't get that job. The Principal had not been happy with me for asking for more money as a permanent substitute. He hired me anyway.

That was my first year as a teacher, the first year I had my own students, students like Joel. Our teacher-student relationship grew and we befriended his parents. We knew that God was a part of their lives but we forgave them this quirk. People said they were part of "that" church. I didn't know what "that" meant. They didn't seem cultish. In fact, they seemed nice, really, really smart, and well grounded. Clearly they had something that we did not.

I remember them telling us that Cassandra would not die. The Lord would not let her. I chuckled at their naiveté despite the seriousness of the situation. Did they not know this disease was the primary genetic killer of children? Did they not know that this very same disease killed my niece? Did they not know that there was no cure? Did they not know what the doctors and everyone else had told us to do? Did they not know that Cassie would soon be too weak to breathe? Did they not know that Cassie would catch pneumonia and die? God would save our daughter? Ha! That was not part of the plan.

Yet, nearly three years later Cassandra lives. She likes to hold hands. She likes to draw with her crayons. She loves to play with her "Little People" house. She loves to stretch her atrophied muscles in the therapy tub. She plays on her computer. She figures out puzzles. She makes her father sing to her every night. She makes her mother keep her on her lap all day. She tries to avoid naps so that she doesn't miss a moment with her mother or father. Her eyes inspire people to give up their time and profit to build her a special home built just for her. She teaches people gratitude and allows them to demonstrate Godly love. Is there anyone who is not profoundly affected by her?

How many miracles has God bestowed upon us? The one where my sister Christy introduced us to Karen who told us about a controversial protocol by a so-called "quack" that could keep her alive? The one where only breaths away from death on Thanksgiving morning she recovered? The one where our God-given strength and wisdom defeated the egoist Harvard doctors to win the fastest insurance appeal (to fly her by private jet away from their incompetence) their business administrator had ever seen? The one where we miraculously found her life-giving nasal prong on a snowy evening in New York while searching for a cure? The one where all the machines failed while she was choking as you had given up? The one that gave you God's grace to endure twenty-two hours a day of intensive care in a solitary room for nearly three years? The one where he miraculously broke the more than twenty years of my afflictions amidst the crushing pressure we were under? The one where no matter how much money we spent on medical equipment and supplies we still had enough to pay living expenses? The one where the entire Cape Cod community unified to improve our quality of life and help build her a custom home? I ask, where has God not provided? In what ways has he not looked over us with indescribable blessing? How has he not taken care of his special creation?

These are merely a handful of minor works the Lord our God has done for us. The real miracles he performed are much more profound. Through Jesus, we have been "blessed beyond the curse and his promise has endured." Reflect back only two years ago. Where were we? I mean besides on a dark path of destruction. We had no sense of meaningful purpose, nothing to hope for, nothing exciting to wake up to. Each day was blandly the same. Where was the expectation that something great might happen each day? That some new insight might be gained? That our daughter might gain strength? That Cassandra would reveal more or herself to us? Was there any wonder about the miraculous beauty of life? Did we ponder how the body makes 3.2 billion proteins and the consequences of missing one peptide of one protein? Look how that missing peptide controls our lives! Did we count each and every breath as a gift from God as we do today?

We were in a state of despair well before Cassandra was even conceived. Our lives remained unfulfilled. Money's promise was an empty idol. Our plan for life had no real meaning. Death was final. Remember when we didn't want children? Why was that? Was it because we thought there was enough misery in the world? Why should we add to it? Yes, I recall what our gift would be. Our legacy was not to add to an already overpopulated, miserable world. Can you imagine the despair it takes to think that way? No wonder we were so upset about the pregnancy test.

Look at what the Lord has done! See how he has changed us: we have faith, we have purpose, we have love, we have each other, we have our daughter, and we have eternal salvation with God. What an incredible concept and comfort. That we, by no merit of our own, have been chosen by God to live eternally with him so long as we honor, obey, and trust in him. And why wouldn't we?

Do you remember how intransigent I was about keeping Cassie alive upon God's revelation that she would live? I questioned the ethics. I questioned God's imparting of grace upon you to fight for her life. Why not let her die in peace. What would be Cassie's quality of life once the Lord preserved her? Was it fair to keep her alive even though she could barely move a finger? Now I see. I questioned God's plan and was shown how very shamefully wrong I was. Now I see that she is and will remain freer than most of humanity. She is free from the evil of the world. She is free from even the witness of evil and its intent. God bestows only goodness upon her. Has he ever allowed anything else? God is with her and she remains unbound by the curses of this world. God gave you sight and wisdom that Cassie shall dance in the freedom of God while she is here and in eternity. If I could fight for even a portion of such grace … but to no avail, for grace is not earned. Grace is freely given by our Father in heaven.

Why then did we fight God even as today? We don't like his plan because it is not ours. Yet looking back, how could it have been any more perfect? Would you trade who Cassie is today for a miracle? What would you do if Cassandra were to stand up, and cast off her medical equipment? I mean long-term. Would you go back to work? What if you found yourself in a windowless cubicle counting numbers for the quarter-end report while daydreaming of days gone by when Cassie was contentedly refusing to nap on your lap? Do you dream of that cubicle today while she gazes into your eyes on your lap? For which of the previous days do you yearn? Take the worst scenario that plays out at least weekly. Cassie plugs and you save her life. What would it be like not to save her life? Is not her life and by extension all life, more precious with each incident? What lesson is God teaching us? Would that each and every person have such a blessing. The world would be God's.

How about a little miracle? How about regaining her smile? I pray for the day that I can see her smile again. I remember how beautiful her smile was and I yearn for it back. Why did she have to lose her smile? It was heartbreaking to see her lose more and more of it. It was inevitably slipping away day by day. What would be lost if she regained her smile? Would her eyes be as expressive as they are today? Why are we forced to discern her countenance and intention? Is this not consistent with God's intention thus far? For without discernment there can be no reflection. There can be no understanding. There can be no wisdom. Even as God does not wholly reveal himself, we receive his wisdom.

The ways in which God has changed us is staggering. Hallelujah, there is no return … yet revealed is God's continued intention and purpose. If there is no return, why has God put it in our hearts to rigorously search and fight for a cure? I fear change, yet with God, I cannot. His promise is too great to ignore. We must continue to obey Him who guides us, for our hope rests in trusting the Lord regardless of where that leads us.

We fasted together in sacrifice and honor to Him as we prayed for his guidance. God promised us both in his own way that he would heal her. He promised you through a dream, and he promised me at the altar. I promised him all glory would go to him. Yet, I wrote to show off the wisdom he had given me instead. He promised he would heal Cassie, not cure the disease or glorify me.

Am I more capable of curing this disease than the scientists and doctors who have advanced degrees, years of research and study, and a lifetime of experience? How could I entertain such foolish folly? I have researched for a year. I can speak the language, yet it means nothing. Just as a body cannot work without a peptide, brains don't mean much without God. Yet captured with the Holy Spirit, all things are possible.

What particular education did we need to follow the path? Other than listen to Christ, what did we do? We followed his light. Should we deviate from that now? Thus, the importance of your dream: your dream is more valuable than all the completed research in the world. Patrick's gift of understanding correctly identified your dream for what it was. Indeed, God will heal Cassie as we heal ourselves. In your dream Cassie enters a pond and emerges with a fish. The fish represents God's desire for her to be raised in a family that lives and feeds upon the Christian faith, a family that prays together in love and unity. We will pray daily for God's intervention in our lives and for his guidance. A family that reads the bible together. A family that takes dominion of Satan through the blood of Christ, daily. We will love and cherish each other as we are God's gift to one another, not merely caretakers of his child. Jesus Christ, our heavenly father, will instruct and bestow upon us direction.

Mary, you have all my love and God's continued grace upon you. You are the one that God has given me to share my love, my hopes, and my dreams. I could ask for no greater gift as God's plan is perfect. Shall we now go forward in love and unity, our destinies irreversibly intertwined with what God has ordained? For better or for worse, we shall honor our commitment to God, ourselves, and each other, and I shall hold your hand through it all, with a grateful heart.

Your loving husband,
Henry

1

Introduction

A. *SPINAL MUSCULAR ATROPHY I*

Spinal Muscular Atrophy (SMA) is a little known and inherited disease that is the number one genetic killer of infants and toddlers.[1] Phenotype (symptoms) results from a homozygous recessive inheritance (meaning that both parents must be carriers).[2] Although there are three or more levels of SMA, this paper concentrates on the most severe form, SMA I.[3]

SMA I is expressed by weakness to the extent that affected infants are described as being "floppy". The weakness is due to the "loss"[4] of alpha motor neurons located in the anterior horn of the spine. Thus, SMA is not a muscular disease but one involving alpha motor neurons. These motor neurons (named "anterior horn cells") control the skeletal (or voluntary) muscles. SMA I infants are unable to raise their heads or sit in an upright position without assistance. They are never able to crawl or walk. The weakness is also proximal more than distal and accompanied by hypotonia.[5] Children are typically diagnosed before the age of six months with onset of phenotype occurring within three months of birth. Without aggressive and rigorous intervention[6], sixty-five percent of those diagnosed usually die before six months and ninety-five percent die before the age of two years.[7] Death typically occurs due to respiratory illness.[8]

Despite its devastating severity, its primary victims, and merciless result, SMA I is relatively unknown to the general population,[9] and much is still unknown about it. Seemingly simple issues, such as whether the disease is progressive, are still the subjects of debate.[10] However, tremendous advancements have been made and there is much optimism that a cure is tantalizingly close.[11]

B. *PROTEIN UPREGULATION METHODOLOGY*

There are nearly 4,000 genetic diseases that afflict human beings. SMA I is among the deadliest. In attempting to conquer such a genetic disease, three questions must be answered:

> (1) What faulty gene causes the disease?[12] In 1995 scientists discovered that the faulty gene for SMA is located on chromosome 5q11 and subsequently named the "Survival of Motor Neuron" gene.
>
> (2) What protein does this gene normally produce? As previously discussed, scientists know that the SMN gene produces SMN protein. SMN protein is critical for the survival of motor neurons. The absence of this protein causes catastrophic consequences, including death (most frequent in SMA I cases).
>
> (2) Can the defective protein or gene be fixed or replaced?[13] This is the question that researchers and scientists are racing to answer by using various methods.

The three primary research fields are: (1) the HDAC inhibitor class of drugs[14] that strive to restore full-length SMN protein production by boosting the output of the backup SMN II gene, (2) gene therapy,[15] and, perhaps most controversially, (3) embryonic stem cells. While each of these treatments holds great potential, they are not without significant hurdles and/or time barriers. Much of the research field is concentrating on HDAC inhibitor drugs to restore full-length SMN protein. Inhibitor drugs are nearest on the horizon of effective treatments, and many clinical trials are underway.[16]

It remains unknown whether or to what extent full-length SMN protein restoration will benefit dead, dying, or underdeveloped motor neurons.[17] Gene therapy holds tremendous promise in the restoration of full-length SMN protein. However, the deaths of patients in the search for cures for other genetic diseases[18] have dealt a significant blow to the field; effective and efficient delivery of genetic therapy poses significant challenges. Lastly, and not withstanding significant national debate, stem cell research remains furthest from reach, although this relatively new field of study continues to make breakthroughs each day.

The challenge of this paper is to decipher under what circumstances and conditions SMA I is treatable using the aforementioned fields or those that warrant further articulation. For example, SMA is not designated as a "pre-screen" disease,[19] yet mounting evidence suggests that the greatest chance of curing this disease lies in its pre- or post-natal prevention.[20] This paper argues that more attention should be given to the apoptotic function of the body and its effects upon motor neurons.[21] Thus, in addition to focusing upon increasing the protein through HDAC inhibitors (after the expression of the disease), controlling protein function (in this case inhibiting the lightning-fast death in SMA I phenotype of motor neurons) may be more immediately fruitful and grant temporary clemency to precious motor neurons while simultaneously altering the patient's genetic code through enriched gene therapy for a sustained remission.[22]

2

Motor Neuron Disease, SMN Protein, and Apoptosis

Motor neuron diseases ("MNDs") are a group of progressive neurological disorders that destroy motor neurons,[23] the nerve cells that control voluntary muscle activities such as speaking, walking, breathing and swallowing. Characteristic symptoms include gradual weakening, wasting away, uncontrollable twitching of the muscles, and stiffness in the arms and legs.[24] Sensation, intellect, memory, and personality are not affected. In some MNDs, such as amyotrophic lateral sclerosis (ALS), muscle weakness is progressive and eventually leads to death when muscles that control breathing are too weak to function. Inherited forms of MNDs are caused by genetic mutations or gene deletions that cause degeneration of motor neurons. There is no cure or standard treatment for MND.[25]

Motor neuron degeneration is also the predominant feature of SMA.[26] Degeneration is specifically of the alpha motor neurons located in the anterior horn of the spine. Death of these cells leads directly to phenotype paralysis in voluntary muscles. While there remain many unanswered questions as to the actual status of the motor neuron cells (are they dead, atrophied, or underdeveloped?), the underlying genetic cause was pinpointed in 1995 to a missing or mutated gene called the SMN gene. The gene is located on chromosomes 5q11 through 5q13. The gene provides instructions for producing SMN protein.[27]

A. *Survival of Motor Neuron Protein and Motor Neurons*

SMN protein is ubiquitous and found in every cell of the body, but the highest levels are found in the spine.[28] For reasons not completely understood, the lack of SMN has a profound adverse effect upon motor neurons that control voluntary muscles (alpha motor neurons).[29] The SMN protein assists in the pre-mRNA processes and may also serve as a Neuronal Apoptotic Inhibitor.[30] The loss of either of these functions within the motor neurons could lead to catastrophic results, including neuronal arrested development, atrophy, or death. Thus, neurodegeneration is a consequence of excessive premature apoptosis (cell suicide) of neurons. Those left surviving have no capacity to regenerate to compensate for the loss.

B. *When Apoptosis Goes Bad*

In SMA I, the loss of motor neurons is rapid, usually within the first three months of life. For this reason, it is critical for newborn diagnosis of SMA. Why a given motor neuron dies at a particular moment in time and how it dies is still not completely known.[31] Whether motor neurons can be protected from death is also the subject of debate. However, scientists speculate that neurons are produced in excess in order that they may compete for contacts with cellular partners and adjust their numbers to provide sufficient innervation of their target muscle groups. This is the most frequent explanation for neuronal death during development.[32] Motor neurons produced in excess compete for access to limited quantities of neurotrophic factors produced by their target neighboring cells. The neurons that are unsuccessful simply die through the apoptotic process.[33] Without the SMN protein, apoptosis may be unregulated and cause massive neuronal suicide.

One possible solution to over-exuberant apoptosis (in the absence of SMN protein) would be to inhibit neuronal apoptosis through the upregulation of neuronal apoptotic inhibitor proteins ("NAIPs")[34]. Indeed, SMN protein is not the only NAIP able to suppress apoptosis. The protein Survivin is also an apoptosis inhibitor/cell-cycle regulator.[35] The upregulation of caspase inhibitors also has been shown to prevent neuronal loss in animal models of head injury and stroke.[36] As with all other current therapies for motor neuron rescue, it is unlikely that anti-apoptotic protein upregulation could occur in a timely enough manner to be of maximum benefit for those suffering from SMA I. However, current technology allows for anti-apoptotic upregulation therapies that could be administered upon phenotype detection.[37] Moreover, in combination with other therapies such as HDAC inhibitors or gene therapy, anti-apoptotic protein upregulation may be of great value.

C. *Unconventional Post-Apoptotic Strategies*

If apoptosis has wreaked its havoc there may be other strategies to pursue such as neuronal regeneration. In humans, during development, there is massive neuronal growth. Once functional connections are made, this growth is shut off by a variety of inhibitory mechanisms that prevent the nervous system from growing out of control. These inhibitors stop nerve cells from growing even after spinal cord injury. Thus, the stop signs that are so important in normal development become a major roadblock to regeneration.[38] The challenge is to remove, go around, or change the stop signs to allow for neuronal regeneration. A small protein named Nogo is part of the "stop sign" (thus the name).[39] Several research groups have generated different mouse models that change the Nogo gene, and the different models show mixed results. For example, some show no regeneration, some show a little regeneration, and some show robust regeneration.[40]

Another challenge to regeneration is to understand how to connect the neurons to the right muscles in order to restore movement. The connections motor neurons make are established during development when newly generated motor neurons in the spinal cord send axons out to "wire" the muscles. During this process, each motor neuron has formed an allegiance to a particular muscle before the axons begin growing.[41] These allegiances are formed by Hox genes that assign muscle targets to all the different motor neurons in the spinal cord. This code generates one hundred different types of motor neurons in the spinal cord. Although not a cure in itself, this important discovery is another piece of a puzzle that adds to the understanding of the basic workings of motor neurons.[42] The better the understanding of the basic workings, the better chance there is of developing regenerative therapies and strategies to restore movement.[43]

Anti-apoptotic agents have the ability to delay the onset of SMA phenotype and/or preserve and restore precious motor neurons. Post-apoptotic strategies promise the future ability to restore motor neurons and movement, even if only on a limited basis. However, these strategies take a back seat to the primary methodology of SMN protein upregulation through SMN1 gene restoration or, more commonly, through its back-up SMN2 gene.

3

Protein Restoration Methods: HDAC Inhibitors, Gene Therapy, and Stem Cells

Humans are the only animals known to carry the SMN2 gene.[44] For this reason, SMA does not naturally occur in nature. Rather, without the SMN1 gene[45], the animal fetus dies in utero. While in humans the SMN2 gene may produce enough full-length SMN protein (averaging approximately ten percent per gene: the more SMN2 genes, the less severe the disease) to maintain the life of a fetus, post-natal levels remain constant and insufficient to maintain healthy motor neurons,[46] thus causing SMA I phenotype and death usually within three to eight months.

Because the severity of the disease is inversely proportionate to the amount of SMN2 protein produced by the SMN2 gene[47] (SMN1 gene is deleted in most cases and nonfunctional in the rest), most therapy targets this gene as a treatment or cure. Although this may seem logical and well conceived, it may not be practical for type I patients. For if severe atrophy is an indication of neuronal death, then no amount of additional full-length protein will bring them back. However, there may be some trophic benefit to the "undead" motor neurons[48]. Thus, a thorough investigation of the primary therapy fields is certainly warranted.

A. *HDAC Inhibitors: Hydroxyurea, Valproic Acid, and Sodium Phenylbutyrate*

Histone deacetylation inhibitors (HDAC inhibitors)[49] are a class of enzymes that many researchers believe is nearest to an effective treatment or cure of SMA. HDAC inhibitors upregulate the production of SMN2 protein. Because only ten percent of the SMN2 protein is useful for neuronal function and survival, upregulation may preserve or protect motor neurons by increasing the levels of useful, full-length protein. If administered during the subacute (pre-symptomatic) phase, they may be able to halt neuronal death and boost the function of those remaining. Given the possibility that many SMA I patients may be experiencing neuronal loss in utero, HDAC inhibitors may have limited effects upon this group. Moreover, when combined with toxicity factors that correlate with the amount necessary to be productive, the length of time for the drugs to take effect, and the speed of neuronal deterioration within SMA I victims, even the most promising results would be limited at best. However, HDAC inhibitors are undoubtedly the nearest of the three fields to a curative therapy for SMA, especially the less severe forms.

i. *hydroxyurea*

Hydroxyurea belongs to a group of medicines called antimetabolites.[50] The drug is used most commonly as a chemotherapy agent in the treatment of cancer.[51] In various studies[52] this drug has been shown to increase the amount of full-length SMN protein in SMA treated cells. Not only were protein levels increased, but intra-nuclear gems (clusters of SMN protein) also were significantly increased in the cells. Pediatric neurologist Dr. Ching Wang of Stanford University is one of the lead investigators of this drug. Wang is the senior author on a research article published in the August 2005 issue of the *Annals of Neurology* that shows the genetic defect can be overcome in human cells.[53] Dr. Wang's team added hydroxyurea to blood cells from five people with type 1 SMA, five with type 2, five with type 3 and five without SMA. His results indicated that the drug was effective at increasing SMN1 in all groups but most dramatically in the SMA-affected cells.

Stunning as this revelation may be, it should be received with guarded reservation. To date, there is no clinical proof that hydroxyurea is a cure or effective treatment for the disease. Some news coverage also appears biased in favor of Wang's[54] experiment as an effective treatment. For example, the article "Denying Death: A Baby-Killing Disease Meets its Match" attributes the ability to speak and the child's longevity to the drug. However, the article minimizes obvious realities that the child requires respiratory assistance.[55] In fact, the only real progress that may be linked to gain from the drug is anecdotal.[56] In a more clinical setting, little more than the number of enrolled patients and the outcome assessment measures (gross motor function measurement, time test and a test for muscle strength known as MUNE) was reported.[57]

Even modest gains are significant but also consistent with the argument that the drug, even when administered at an early age, may sustain those motor neurons that remain. However, this was not apparent in our own daughter.[58] In over a year on the drug, we have noticed a slight increase in strength in her left arm and shoulder concurrent with an intentional three-ounce weight reduction.[59] The results we were anticipating were not realized, yet we dare not remove her from the drug for fear of further deterioration.

ii. *Valproic (Valproate) Acid*

Valproic acid is most commonly used as an anticonvulsant in the treatment of epilepsy and as a mood-stabilizing drug for bipolar disorder. It is also used in the treatment of migraine headaches and schizophrenia. A 2005 study also revealed that the drug (an inhibitor of the enzyme histone deacetylase 1) when treating AIDS in tandem with highly active antiretroviral therapy (HAART) showed a 75% reduction in latent HIV infection.[60] Because valproic acid is an HDAC inhibitor, well-tolerated[61], and FDA approved (on the market as Depakote for decades)[62], it appears to be a perfect candidate as a trial drug.

Valproic Acid has demonstrated effectiveness in increasing levels of SMN protein by up to four times in one study[63]. In an earlier 2004 study of cultured cells, the drug also increased production of SMN1 protein. The optimistic article (while cautioning that it is too soon to know whether the drug will have therapeutic effects in humans) even suggests that these findings may "halt or reverse the course of this devastating disease."[64] Indeed, valproic acid would appear most promising to those who suffer from lesser forms of the disease. This is because they lose their motor neurons less rapidly (as evidenced by a more gradual loss of motor function).

While these findings are indeed promising, some hurdles still need to be cleared, especially for children suffering from SMA I. For example, because liver toxicity is especially prevalent for children under two (NINDS), the amount necessary for therapeutic value may prohibit those who need it most. As previously seen, most infants and toddlers with this form of the disease die within the first six to eight months. Survivors rapidly lose motor function resulting from the loss of motor neurons. Waiting until after the age of two (or even one) may exclude them from therapeutic gain.[65]

iii. *Sodium Phenylbutyrate*

Sodium phenylbutyrate (SB) is used to treat a deficiency of enzymes that help remove ammonia from the body (Medline Plus 3).[66] SB also is being studied in the treatment of neurological disorders such as Huntington's disease and as a cancer chemotherapy agent.[67] SB, like valproic acid, has been in clinical trials with confirmed type II patients (age range 2.6-12.7).[68] Researchers found "significant increases in the scores of Hammersmith functional scale between the baseline …"[69] One of the most positive aspects of this drug is its tolerability.[70] The butyrate drugs also have been the best clinically-studied compounds and are known to readily reach and penetrate the blood-barrier of the brain (Neals ALS Clinical trials). Perhaps most strikingly, what separates SB from other HDAC inhibitors is its anti-apoptotic potential. MDA researchers discovered that SB appears to interfere with a cell death program and extends the lives of mice with amyotrophic lateral sclerosis[71]. Tolerability, effective targeting, and anti-apoptotic features make SB the best therapeutic drug for SMA I patients and for those patients under the age of two.[72] Not only could it upregulate SMN protein without significant side effects, but most importantly, it preserved precious motor neurons. For these reasons, further investigation into this drug is warranted.

HDAC inhibitors are the most immediate of the promising therapies on the horizon. However, it appears as though the lesser SMAs will benefit the most, primarily because of rapid neuronal loss in SMA I. Thus, without early intervention such as newborn screening, it is unlikely that significant arrest of SMA phenotype could occur. Without newborn screening or some other mechanism for early detections, it is unlikely that parents would have any idea that a deadly disease is taking its course in their child. By the time of diagnosis, acceptance, and reaction, much of the neuronal damage will have already taken place. However, HDAC inhibitors (especially those with anti-apoptotic qualities) may possess the limited ability to boost the function of remaining motor neurons and halt some neuronal loss, even in SMA I patients. In the near future it is very possible that newborn screening for SMA will become law. Should this happen, HDAC inhibitors in conjunction with apoptotic inhibitors would be a promising combination to halt the disease in its tracks.

B. *GENE THERAPY*

Gene therapy is a relatively new frontier[73] aimed at treating human disease by the transfer of genetic material into specific cells of a patient in order to replace a defective gene or to introduce a new function to the cell.[74] While in theory gene therapy may seem promising, many problems persist, and recent deaths have forced researchers to rethink their methodology. Researchers face daunting challenges. For example, a correct copy of the gene must be available, the specific cells in the body requiring treatment must be identified and accessible, and a means of efficiently delivering correct copies of the gene to these cells must also be available in such a way that the gene can penetrate the body's defense mechanisms and be expressed at the appropriate level for a sufficient duration.[75] Of these challenges, "gene delivery" looms largest.[76]

i. *Viral Vectors*

One of the most promising DNA delivery systems is found in nature in the form of viruses.[77] Viruses attack their hosts and introduce their genetic material into the host cell as part of their replication cycle. This genetic material contains basic 'instructions' on how to produce more copies of these viruses, hijacking the body's normal production machinery to serve the needs of the virus. The host cell carries these new instructions and produces additional copies of the virus, leading to more and more cells becoming infected. Scientists have realized that viruses can be used as vehicles to carry "good" genes into a human cell.[78] Re-engineered viruses[79] are called viral vectors. Because the viruses can no longer produce their parent virus, they are safe delivery mechanisms. Of course, numerous problems present with this oversimplification. Notwithstanding ethical considerations[80] and undesired effects (such as cancer), 'infecting' the correct target cell in the body and ensuring that the inserted gene does not disrupt any vital genes already within the genome are all significant challenges that molecular biologists face.[81]

ii. *Great Success and Tragic Results*

Dr. W. French Anderson[82] presided over the first experimental gene therapy treatment of a human in 1990. The patient, then-four-year-old Ashanti DeSilva suffered from a condition known as severe combined immune deficiency (SCID) caused by a defective gene.[83] To cure her, Anderson and his colleagues took healthy copies of those genes[84] and injected them into viruses engineered to serve as genetic carrying messengers; then they transferred the viruses into DeSilva's body. The phenomenal success led to a media frenzy that hailed gene therapy as a breakthrough in the treatment of genetic disorders (*Gene Therapy* 1999). Then in September of 1999 eighteen year-old Jesse Gelsinger died after undergoing gene therapy for a rare metabolic disorder at the University of Pennsylvania Medical Center.[85] This would not be the only time that the safety and effectiveness of gene therapy had been called into question. Subsequent gene therapy trials after DeSilva's case failed to reverse the disease.[86] In April of 2000 *Science Magazine* presented two cases of SCID treated by gene therapy. The cells appeared to be working and the therapy appeared successful. In all, ten SCID patients were treated in the trial. In a subsequent October 2003 article in *Science Magazine* two boys undergoing the treatment had developed a form of T-cell proliferation similar to leukemia,[87] and SCID gene therapy trials were put on hold worldwide.[88]

iii. *Gene Therapy Strategies for SMA*

The primary strategy for correction of SMA through gene therapy is to restore SMN gene protein output. In 2003 an adenovirus-mediated gene showed that SMN could be efficiently expressed in patient fibroblasts (skin cells).[89] This therapy led to the restoration of nuclear gems (absent in patients with severe SMA) that are thought to be a critical part of SMA restoration.[90] This work was the first demonstration that virus-based delivery of SMN-coding gene could restore the normal SMN expression pattern in SMA patient-derived cells and therefore be a potential long-term therapy for the disease.[91] However, like HDAC inhibitors, this study focuses on protein restoration at the expense of ignoring the status of motor neurons. For example, in 1999 researchers studied the effectiveness of gene transfer of inhibitors of apoptotic proteins (IAPs). Specifically, they investigated the ability of IAP genes in a neuronal model of apoptosis. Forced expression of IAPs blocked apoptotic activity and reduced DNA fragmentation.[92] Even though neurons were only protected from apoptosis for twenty-four hours, the study was important for continuation of research in the field of neuronal apoptotic suppression gene therapy. A 2004 gene therapy study (that may be the most exciting breakthrough for the SMA community) built on the idea of simultaneous motor neuron preservation and upregulation SMN protein levels.

In 2004 gene therapy researchers at Oxford Biomedica[93] considered how to deliver SMN to keep motor neurons alive. In response, they developed a transfer system (lentivector) to deliver genes to neurons. Their particular viral vector led to long-term correction of amyotrophic lateral sclerosis (ALS) in a mouse model for over five months.[94] Similarly, the Lentivector-mediated SMN gene therapy in SMA mice improved motor neuron survival and induced a small but still significant increase in survival.[95] The results of the study stress the importance of gene therapy expression of SMN at the onset of disease. If it can be translated to humans, it would mean an extension in life span and a delay in the motor phenotype of severe SMA.[96] Lastly, this study is critical because it stresses the immediacy of motor neuron rescue. The study indicates that delivery of therapeutic candidates in the vicinity of degenerating motor neurons is critical to maximize rescue efficiency.

Realistically, the recurrent problem of early detection and rapid neuronal deterioration omits the possibility of maximum motor neuron rescue for SMA I victims. Although, there may be some benefit such as functional boost to remaining neurons, the risks associated with the treatment may not be worth a benefit that likely would not surpass that of the less risky HDAC inhibitor therapies.

C. *Stem Cells*

Emerging stem cell technology is perhaps the most exciting, controversial, and distant of therapies. The promise of cures of incurable diseases distantly lies within this field. That is because stem cells have the ability to transform into a dazzling array of specialized cells that comprise the human body.[97] They may be just the keys that unlock the mysteries of human disease. They have the potential to treat the most serious medical conditions such as cancer and birth defects, restore cells and tissues, and even grow organs.[98] The most controversial of these therapies, human embryonic stem cells (hESCs), have yet to fulfill their expectations. Scientists have done little more than experiment with hESCs since 1998.[99] In fact, it is adult stem cells (ASCs) that have thus far proven themselves most useful. Doctors have been transferring ASCs in bone marrow transplants for over forty years. More advanced techniques of collecting or "harvesting" ASCs are now used in order to treat leukemia, lymphoma, several inherited blood disorders, diabetes, and advanced kidney cancer.[100]

Even within this field, a cure for SMA I may remain elusive for the foreseeable future. As this paper has indicated throughout, the greatest challenge for SMA I therapy is early intervention. Without it, the motor neurons are lost. Although many therapies promise to realistically boost or enhance the function of remaining neurons, a complete cure would rest in the ability to create new or regenerated neurons. However, stem cells offer a great deal more than merely a neuronal boost.

i. *Adult Stem Cells (ASCs)*

ASCs are undifferentiated (unspecialized) cells that are found in a differentiated (specialized) tissue in the adult, such as blood. Generally, ASCs differentiate into the specialized cell types of the tissue from which it originated[101] and for this reason they are known as multi-potent stem cells. ASCs are found in places such as bone marrow (where adult hematopoietic stem cells are found) that are capable of developing into blood and immune cells.[102] Recently, scientists reported that under certain conditions these same stem cells also could develop into cells that have many of the characteristics of neurons.[103] Other types of ASCs include endothelial stem cells that form along the vascular system (arteries and veins) and mesenchymal stem cells from bone, cartilage, muscle, and fat.[104] ASCs can also be found in the brain (neural stem cells),[105] retina of the eye, skeletal muscle, dental pulp, liver, skin, the lining of the gastrointestinal tract, and pancreas. Although ASCs have not proven to be pluripotent,[106] they have been shown to be capable of developing into cells from all three embryonic germ layers.[107] Interestingly, adult stem cells from bone marrow generated cells that resemble neurons and other types are found in the brain. Thus, ASCs have the potential to develop into all three embryonic germ layers and offer an alternative to controversial hESCs for those suffering from incurable, catastrophic, or chronic diseases and afflictions. However, there are significant hurtles to this endeavor. For example, adult stem cells are rare. Often they are difficult to identify, isolate, purify, and proliferate. In order to use adult stem cells for cell-replacement strategies, researchers must overcome the insufficient numbers of cells available for transplantation. This is because most ASCs, when grown in a culture dish, are unable to proliferate in an unspecialized state for long periods of time.[108] In cases where they can be grown and proliferate, researchers have not been able to direct them to become specialized as functionally useful cells.[109] To offset this problem, scientists have been highly creative. Researchers in the August 26, 2005 issue of *Science* reported fusing an adult skin cell with an embryonic stem cell and showing that the cell was reprogrammed to its embryonic state.[110] This is particularly exciting for two reasons: (1) the stem cells have a greater chance of being accepted by the body, and (2) the hybrid cells could theoretically be used to produce embryonic stem cell lines that are tailored to individual patients without the need to create and destroy human embryos.[111]

ii. *Younger Stem Cells: Umbilical Cord Stem Cells*

Stem cells derived from umbilical cord blood or from the pulp under baby teeth are "younger" stem cells than those obtained from adults. They are able to divide for longer times in cell cultures than most adult stem cells and may give rise to different tissues as well. Primarily, umbilical cord blood stem cells are used in patients that have been irradiated or treated with specific drugs for cancer or leukemia to reconstitute blood cell formation.[112] It is an alternative to bone marrow collection as a source of donor hematopoietic stem cells from which new, healthy blood can be produced.

Umbilical cord blood stem cells (UCBSCs) are now being researched for treatment in other diseases such as Krabbe disease,[113] adrenoleukodystrophy (ALD),[114] and amyotrophic lateral sclerosis (ALS),[115] despite scientific disagreement as to UCBSC effectiveness. For example, the research team at Families of Spinal Muscular Atrophy Research (FSMA) acknowledge that although UCBSCs can turn into cartilage, muscle and blood (and be useful in the treatment of lymphoma and leukemia), they concur that the therapy would be ineffective for producing motor neurons.[116] Yet, in 2005 University of North Carolina researchers conducted a study of the effects of cord blood transplantation on newborns and infants with Krabbe disease (a lethal disease due to the lack of an enzyme called GALC that breaks down important compounds in the body). All of the treated newborns showed normal neurological development after the transplantation, except for their motor skills. The older infants had minimal neurological improvement, and their survival rate was no better than that of untreated children. Clearly, this case study supports the premise of early treatment of neurological disease but adds to the debate about the effectiveness of varying stem cell therapies.

Notwithstanding effectiveness, mounting concern over safety is a major part of UCBSC debate, specifically, how the body will react to foreign bodies. To perform a UCBSC transplant, the immune system must be repressed to avoid an adverse reaction. Immunorepression can lead to other complications due to pathogenic exposure. Methodologies such as preimplantation genetic diagnosis (PGD) can mitigate the immune system risk of cord blood stem cell transfer, although not without ethical controversy within its own domain.[117]

An alternative to PGD, but no less controversial, is for fertility clinics to perform the PGD to detect for the genetic disease and: (1) remove the single cell as usual, (2) allow it to divide into two cells, (3) use one of the cells to test for genetic problems, and (4) use the other cell to establish a stem cell line that could be used (in the case of SMA) to create embryonic stem cells lines (that could differentiate into motor neurons) without killing the embryo.[118] Although there are many questions regarding the ethics and efficacy of such methods, the use of UCBSCs should not be readily overlooked as new methodologies and technologies seem to emerge almost daily.

iii. *Human Embryonic Stem Cells (hESCs)*

An embryonic stem cell is derived from a group of cells called the inner cell mass, which is part of the early (4-5 day) embryo called the blastocyst. Once removed from the blastocyst, the cells of the inner cell mass can be cultured into embryonic stem cells. Once this is done, the embryo is destroyed.[119] The cells are considered pluripotent because they have the ability to give rise to types of cells that develop from the three germ layers (mesoderm, endoderm, and ectoderm) from which all the cells of the body arise.[120] The cells divide continuously in tissue culture dishes in an incubator, but at the same time they maintain the ability to generate any cell type when placed into the correct environment to cause their differentiation.[121]

The most publicized use for stem cells is their ability to form different types of cells that can be used to restore or replace damaged tissue in patients with disease or injury. Although tissue replacement has not yet been done on humans, significant advances have been made in the laboratory. For example, in 2000 scientists at Johns Hopkins reported that they restored movement to newly paralyzed rodents by injecting stem cells into the animals' spinal fluid.[122] Researchers speculate that "fewer nerve cells are needed for the function of muscles than they originally expected." Scientists also theorized that "stem cells haven't restored the nerve cell-to-muscle units required for movement but that they protect or stimulate the few undamaged nerve cells that still remain." Although the experiment was done with embryonic stem cells, the same theory of motor neurons may hold true for other types of treatments including HDAC inhibitors, gene therapy, and adult stem cell therapies. In 2006, leading hESC researcher Dr. Douglas Kerr and his colleagues showed that new functional motor neuron circuits can be created by injecting motor neurons derived from mouse embryonic stem cells into the spinal cord of animals. These new connections partially restored function in paralyzed rats by creating neuron connections from the spinal cord to the muscles.[123] The youngest SMA Type I patients would be particularly amenable to this type of therapy because patients are usually infants still in developmental stages.[124]

iv. *Neural Stem Cells and Motor Neurons*

Because there is not yet an effective treatment that prevents the onset of motor neuron disease, one focus (and a focus of this paper) is to restore the function of the motor neurons before and/or as they start to degenerate. The focus within this field is treatment with embryonic and/or neural stem cells.[125] Dr. Evan Snyder of Harvard University (in conjunction with Boston Children's Hospital) transplanted cloned human neural stem cells derived from a fifteen-week-old aborted human fetus.[126] Their experiments demonstrate that these neural stem cells can replace missing or deficient brain cells.[127] Leaving ethical concerns aside, it remains unanswered whether older animals will benefit from transplantation as younger animals have. And: can transplanted cells survive an ongoing degenerative disease process, or will they fall victim to degeneration, as have their predecessors?[128] Regardless of the type of stem cells, and even though it is still not fully understood how stem cells exert their effects,[129] stem cells have had promising results in the repair of damaged motor neurons in mice. Despite the significant challenge of repairing motor neurons in mice, this prospect is even a greater task in humans.[130] Thus, using stem cells to replace dying and dead motor neurons is a colossal task. Perhaps more practical would be to improve the health of cells near motor neurons to extend their life.[131] In cases of SMA I where significant damage has already occurred, non-embryonic stem cells may still be useful to boost the function of the surviving motor neurons to a greater degree, or in conjunction with, HDAC inhibitors or gene therapy.

4

Combination Therapies

One of the most exciting research areas is the development of combination therapies that can take the best ideas of several fields and combine them to make an effective strategy for recovery. One such strategy combines stem cell and gene therapy. The process includes isolating stem cells (such as bone marrow or muscle), growing them in the lab, treating them with therapeutic genes, and then returning them to affected areas where they become "normal".[132] Dr. Louis Kunkel (of Boston Children's Hospital)[133] separated stem cells from healthy muscle tissue, injected them into previously destroyed bone marrow, and found that the transplanted muscle stem cells not only regenerated the recipient's bone marrow, but also contributed to the recipient mouse's voluntary muscle. Because the stem cells were originally isolated from a healthy mouse, the new muscle cells had full functional genes for dystrophin (the protein missing in Duchenne dystrophy).[134] Fellow researcher Margaret Goodell (Baylor College of Medicine in Houston) applied her stem cell purification procedure and theorized that the best therapy option would be to take someone's own stem cells from bone marrow or muscle, treat the affected area with traditional gene therapy to correct the problem, and then transplant the re-engineered cells into the body.

To apply this theory to SMA I, one might (1) create and/or extract neural (or similar type) stem cells from a diseased patient (with SMN protein deficiency), (2) add the SMN1 gene so that the cells produce SMN protein, and (3) transplant the re-engineered cells into the affected area (anterior horn of spine). The anticipated outcome might include increased SMN protein production, neurotrophic benefit for existing motor neurons, and boosting the strength of existing motor neurons. One might also add specific genes that induce neuronal growth or genes that upregulate neuronal growth.[135] The re-engineered cells could be turned on or off or "instructed" to increase or decrease the amount of therapeutic output through administered drugs. The intent would be to create "super motor neurons" out of the surviving neurons, strengthen them, and allow them to grow.

There are some profound advantages to this therapy: (1) the addition of the therapeutic transgene to the delivery cells takes place outside the patient, which allows researchers an important measure of control,[136] and (2) investigators can genetically engineer or "program" the cells' level and rate of production of the therapeutic agent.[137] Although hematopoietic stem cells have been a delivery cell of choice, neural stem cells (converted from adult stem cells such as from the marrow) have been used. Myoblasts (muscle stem cells) also may be good candidates for stem cell gene therapy because the therapeutic agents produced by the transgene area are accessible to nerves.[138]

Proof of this principle rests in an animal study of myoblast (muscle tissue) mediated gene transfer involving a mouse model of familial ALS.[139] However (like most experiments discussed in this paper), it was performed before the death of the motor neurons. Therefore it does not properly address whether it could be of value in the restoration of the motor neurons.[140] It should also be noted that no consistent therapeutic effects have been achieved in gene therapy trials to date.[141] In principle at least, the use of human embryonic stem cells might overcome limitations.[142]

An important feature of the optimal cell for delivering a therapeutic transgene would be its ability to retain the therapeutic transgene even as it proliferates or differentiates into specialized cells. Most of the cell-based gene therapies attempted so far have used viral vehicles to introduce the transgene into the hematopoietic stem cell. Another way to accomplish this is to insert the therapeutic transgene into one of the chromosomes of the stem cell.[143]

Achieving clinical success with cell-based gene therapy will require new knowledge and advances in several key areas including the design of viral and nonviral vehicles for introducing therapeutic agents into cells, the ability to direct where in a cell the transgene is introduced, the ability to direct the genetically modified stem cells, regulation of the production of the therapeutic agent within the stem cell, and management of immune reactions to the gene therapy process. These obstacles should not automatically rule out further investigation of these new methodologies.

A. *Gene and Stem Cell Therapy in Autoimmune Diseases*

SMA does not fit the criteria of autoimmune disease[144] or muscular dystrophy.[145] However, just as researchers are studying therapies for SMA as they would muscular dystrophies, so should they search for therapies as though it were an autoimmune disease. Currently there is an extensive amount of cell-based gene therapy research being conducted in animal models of autoimmune disease, the goal being to modify the aberrant, inflammatory immune response that is characteristic of autoimmune diseases.[146] In the same way, gene and stem cell therapies should be used to block apoptotic processes that destroy the motor neurons. For example, in severe SMA, dysfunctional neuronal apoptotic inhibitor proteins are unable to correctly read DNA,[147] thus permitting unopposed developmental apoptosis to occur in sensory and motor systems that result in lethal muscular atrophy. Transferring a gene that encodes for anti-caspase 3 activation[148] could redirect and regulate the apoptotic processes to a more "tolerant" state, thus delaying or halting motor neuron destruction. Even less complicated would be to transfer genetic material into the slowly dividing stem cells to produce the intended apoptotic inhibitor protein at levels that can be controlled. While these methods may halt motor neuron destruction, they still do not address the core issue of SMN protein deficiency within the motor neuron axons. Without this protein, the axon cells may trigger the suicide code. This may indicate a need to elongate the truncated SMN protein using HDAC inhibitor drugs (or other means as described herein).

5

Emerging Therapies

A. *OLIGONUCLEOTIDES*

Many genetic diseases are caused by the mutation of just one or two of the 3.2 billion base pairs of DNA that comprise the human genome. Many of these mutations occur on the intron (meaningless DNA code). However, when a mutation occurs on the exon (important DNA code), it may adversely affect splicing[149] and fatal consequences may result. SMA is a genetic disease that arises from a deletion and/or mutation of the SMN1 gene that causes the body to rely on the faulty SMN2. The SMN2 gene contains a lesion at exon seven, which causes it to be "skipped" during pre-mRNA transcription. The result is a non-functional, truncated protein. About ten percent of the protein is useful, full-length protein. Scientists are therefore concentrating on boosting the output of the SMN2 protein production through the use of HDAC inhibitors.

Another approach would be to prevent the exon from being "skipped" during pre-mRNA transcription. The prevention of exon skipping would have the effect of producing the vital full-length protein that is essential for motor neuron and axonal growth. One way of preventing exon skipping is through the use of oligonucleotides.[150] The idea is to make short pieces of oligos that would stick to a target exon (such as exon 7) by attaching another piece of RNA that carries good signals for splicing. This would mean that good signals could be stuck onto RNA that had poor signals. An experiment was successfully attempted on SMA-affected tissue in vitro (test tubes) that showed that the oligo would stimulate splicing in exon seven (which is normally skipped). This experiment showed that some of the cells were able to produce enough of the protein for it to accumulate as normal in spots in the nucleus. The next immediate goal of the team is to find a way of making the oligos that will allow them to work well and safely in animals with SMA and, ultimately, in humans.[151]

6

Conclusions

Never in human history has there been such curative knowledge, technology, and opportunity. If ever there was hope to cure an incurable disease, it is now. Even so, challenges within the field of neurodegeneration are great. While SMA I appears to be relatively straightforward as a single-gene mutation, the consequences of its absence are perhaps greater than expected for SMA I sufferers.

Spinal Muscular Atrophy is a disease that attacks motor neurons due to a lack of survival of motor neuron protein produced by the SMN1 gene. SMA victims are deleted for this gene, or (less commonly) it is mutated. Humans possess a backup SMN2 gene that produces approximately ten percent of the useful, full-length protein. Thus, researchers, scientists, and doctors are concentrating on protein upregulation of the SMN2 gene or replacing the SMN1 gene. Protein upregulation strategies hold much promise for the lesser SMAs as neuronal deterioration is slower in these patients. Evidence suggests that the most opportune time to halt or reverse the disease is with early or subacute phenotype. Thus, there is significantly more opportunity for neuronal rescue for the lesser SMAs and a greater chance of recovery.

That does not mean protein upregulation will be an ineffective treatment for SMA I. If early detection mechanisms are implemented (such as newborn screening), protein upregulation would be a powerful therapy. Even so, the speed of neuronal death is so fast and so early that it may render the singular protein upregulation strategy inefficient and insufficient for significant recovery in SMA I sufferers. For example, dosage levels of therapeutic upregulators may be prohibitive for newborns and infants: the amount of time the therapy takes to begin SMN protein restoration or an adverse reaction to the therapeutic agent may influence the degree of recovery. For this reason, therapies such as apoptotic inhibitors, neurotrophic protection agents, and/or hormonal interventions (such as decreasing testosterone levels) should be considered in tandem with protein upregulators.

Currently, at the time of SMA I diagnosis, most parents are told to enjoy the time they have left with their child. There is no attempt to begin any therapy to preserve motor neurons when they need it most. Even if protein upregulator strategies are not possible, neuroprotection and hormonal intervention to halt, delay, or diminish progression severity are not outside the realm of technological capability and should actively be pursued. Moreover, for sufferers who have surpassed the generally accepted window of early opportunity (three months or less) and who survive the disease phenotype, other types of therapies that concentrate on rehabilitation of the motor neurons are necessary.

The most difficult aspect of curing SMA I is undoubtedly motor neuron restoration. Despite promising developments of creating a working neuron for a mouse through the use of eHSCs, much more experimentation and research will be necessary before this can be applied to humans. Moreover, ethical concerns also may pose a barrier to this type of technology. Research into combination stem and gene therapy is a promising lead that is no further off in the distance than new stem cell motor neuron. In fact, it may even be more technologically relevant to re-engineer the surviving motor neurons to create "super strength" neurons that would not only boost gross motor function but sprout new axonal growth.

The most significant opportunity to survive and treat SMA I is early detection. Incredibly, the number one genetic killer of babies and infants does not even make the original list of eighty-four diseases and disorders considered for inclusion of newborn screening. This is tantamount to allowing a known child killer to snatch babies from the homes of unsuspecting parents, slowly suffocate them until death, and search for more victims without impunity. It should not and cannot be allowed. Many organizations such as Families of Spinal Muscular Atrophy and fightsma.org are working hard to gain the vital "newborn screening" status. The researchers also are doing their part to solve this complex puzzle. Enhancing community awareness, petitioning politicians, and raising funds are actions that all who have been affected can take to cure this despicable disease.

Bibliography

"AAAS." Reprogramming Adult Stem Cells. News Archives Aug. 2005 <www.aaas.org/news>.

"About." Cord Blood Transplantation Affects Progression of Krabbe Disease. Rare/Orphan Diseases 2006 <www.rarediseases.about.com>.

Acharya, Sanjukta. "RxPG News Muscular Dystrophies Channel." Valproate Effective in Adult Spinal Muscular Atrophy. RxPG News Jun. 2006 <www.rxpgnews.com>.

Ackerman, Todd. "Chron.com." Scientists See Value in Both Embryonic, Adult Stem Cells Houston and Texas: Jul. 2006 <www.chron.com>.

Associated Press. "Closer to a Cure." Cape Cod Times 1 Sept. 2006:2.

Azzouz, Mimoun et al. "Lentivector-Mediated SMN Replacement in a Mouse Model of Spinal Muscular Atrophy" Journal of Clinical Investigation. 114(2004):1726.

Bach, John R. Management of Patients with Neuromuscular Disease. Philadelphia: Hanley & Belfus Inc. 2004.

BBC News. Self-Repair Gene Therapy Promise. BBC News May 2006. May 2006 <www.news.bbc.com>.

Biomedica. Oxford Biomedica Publishes Preclinical Efficacy Results with its Product Candidate SMN1-G for Spinal Muscular Atrophy Oxford Biomedica Dec. 2004. Jul. 2006 <www.biomedica-usa.com>.

Biomedica. MoNuDin: A Gene-Based Therapeutic for Motor Neuron Disease Product Profile Sep. 2005. Jul. 2006 <www.biomedica-usa.com>.

Binhai Zheng. "Roman Reed Program Research Grants." Functional Analysis of Nogo in CNS Axon Regeneration Using a Nogo Null Mutant RRPRG 2005. Feb. 2006.

Brown, Stuart F. "Mindfully." Building DNA Chips Using Tricks from Nanotech and Bioinformatics Soul of New Gene Machines: May 2005. Jul. 2006 <www.mindfully.org>.

Buss, Robert R. et al. Annual Reviews. "Adaptive Roles of Programmed Cell Death During Nervous System Development" Mar. 2006. Jul. 2006.

Cartegni, Krainer. "NCBI PubMed" Correction of Disease-Associated Exon Skipping by Synthetic Exon-Specific Activators. NCBI PubMed Abstract Feb. 2003. Jul. 2006.

CBC News. Valproate Helped People with SMA Get Stronger. CBC News Jun. 2006.

Cell Transplants International LLC. Frequently Asked Questions. celltherapy.com 2002 <www.celltherapy.com>.

Center for Genetics Education. Genes and Chromosomes. Center for Genetics Education 2006 <www.genetics.com>.

Center for Genetics Education. Genes Therapy: Genes and Health Feb. 2004 <www.genetics.com>.

Children's Hospital Boston. MRRC Project(s). The Snyder Laboratory 2006 <www.childrenshopital.org>.

Cocco, Melanie. "Roman Reed Program Research Grants." Structure of Proteins That Inhibit CNS Repair: Nogo and its Receptor. RRPRG 2005.

Conger, Krista. "Stanford School of Medicine" Drug Provides Glimmer of Hope for Children Suffering Fatal Genetic Disease. Stanford Oct. 2005 <www.mednews.stanford.edu>.

Conger, Krista. "Stanford School of Medicine" Denying Death: A Baby-Killing Disease Meets its Match. Stanford Spring 2006. Aug. 2006 <www.mednews.stanford.edu>.

Critpath.org. Cell Suicide in Health and Disease. Scientific American Dec. 1996. Jul. 2006 <www.critpath.org>.

Cromie, William J. "The Harvard University Gazette." Nerve Cell Clones Repair Brain Damage. Harvard Gazetteer Archives: Jan. 1999 <www.hno.harvard.edu/gazette>.

Cure Paralysis NOW Advocacy Group. What is an Embryonic Stem Cell (ESC)? Cure Paralysis Now May 2003 <www.cureparalysisnow.org>

Darras, Dr. "Scientific Research Update." From the Desk of Dr. Darras Aug. 2006.

DeVivo, Dr. Darryl. "Columbia University Medical Center: INVIVO" Scientists Crack Neuron Code Jan. 2006.

Dentzer, Susan. "Online NewsHour." Online Focus: Gene Therapy Dec. 1999. Jul. 2006 <www.pbs.org/newshour>.

DiDonato, C.J. et al. "NCBI/PubMed." abstract Development of a Gene Therapy Strategy for the Restoration of Survival Motor Neuron Protein Expression: Implications for Spinal Muscular Atrophy PubMed Jan. 2003. Jul. 2006 <www.ncbi.nlm.nih.gov/entrez>

Dreyfus, Gideon. "Howard Hughes Medical Institute" Ribonucleoprotein Complexes: Assembly, Function, and Roles in Human Disease. HHMI Jan. 2006. Jul 2006 <www.hhmi.org/research/investigators/dreyfuss.html>.

Families of Spinal Muscular Atrophy. Transcript of Q&A FSMA Research 2005. Jan. 2006 <www.fsma.org>.

FSMA. Stem Cells For the Treatment of SMA Research: Winter 2005/06 <www.fsma.org>.

Fight SMA: Fact Sheet. FightSMA: Accelerating a Cure for Spinal Muscular Atrophy. Aug. 2006 <www.fightsma.com>.

Fight SMA Research News 2004. Jul. 2005 <www.fightsma.com/Darryl_DeVivo>.

Genetics Home Reference. SMN1. Genetics Home Reference Jul. 2006 <www.ghr.nlm.nih.gov>.

Gorman, Jessica. "Science News." Delivering the Goods: Gene Therapy Without the Virus Jan. 2003 <www.sciencenews.org>.

Grzeschik, Susanna M. et al. "Wiley Interscience." Hydroxyurea Enhances SMN2 Gene Expression in Spinal Muscular Atrophy Cells. Abstract, Wiley Interscience Jul. 2005. Jul. 2006 <www3.interscience.wiley.com>.

Herrera-Sot, Jose. Spinal Muscular Atrophy. Oct. 2004 <www.emedicine.com>.

Hertel, Klemens. Abstract: "Correction of SMN2 Pre-mRNA Splicing by Antisense U7 Small Nuclear RNAs" Families of Spinal Muscular Atrophy 15(2006):1.

Hirtz, D. Challenges and Opportunities in Clinical Trials for Spinal Muscular Atrophy. Neurology. 2005. 2006 <www.neurology.com>.

Hopkins Medicine. Stem Cells Graft in Spinal Cord Restore Movement in Paralyzed Mice Hopkins Medicine Nov. 2000 <www.hopkinsmedicine.org>.

Irwin, Joseph et al. "Families of Spinal Muscular Atrophy" Abstract: SMA Research Update from the Families of SMA Supported Research Meeting. FSMA Aug. 2006 <www.curesma.org>.

Jablonka, Sibylle. "Wiley Interscience" Axonal Defects in Mouse Models of Motoneuron Disease. Wiley Interscience Abstract Dec. 2003. Jul. 2006 <www3.interscience.wiley.com>.

Jones, Kevin et al. "JBC Online" Direct Interaction of the Spinal Muscular Atrophy Disease Protein SMN with the Small Nucleolar RNA-Associated Protein Fibrillarin. JBC Online Abstract Aug. 2001 <www.jbc.org>.

Journal of Nature. May 2004, Volume 429, Issue 6990, pp. 413-17.

Katsuno, Masahisa et al. "ScienceDirect." Testosterone Reduction Prevents Phenotypic Expression in a Transgenic Mouse Model of Spinal and Bulbar Muscular Atrophy Neuron (35) Aug. 2002 <www.sciencedirect.com/science>.

Kerr, Douglas A. et al. “Proceedings of the National Academy of Sciences of the United States of America.” Abstract Survival Motor Neuron Protein Modulates Neuron-Specific Apoptosis. PNAS Nov. 2000. Jul. 2006 <www.pnas.org>.

Lewis, Ricki. “The Scientist.” Preimplantation Genetic Diagnosis: The Next Big Thing? Research Nov. 2000 <www.the-scientist.com>.

Lindsay, RM. “NCBI PubMed” Trophic Protection of Motor Neurons: Clinical Potential in Motor Neuron Diseases. NCBI PubMed Abstract Dec. 1994 <www.ncbi.nlm.nih.gov/entrez>.

Liston, P. et al. “NCBI PubMed” Suppression of Apoptosis in Mammalian Cells by NAIP and a Related Family of IAP Genes. Nature Abstract Jan. 1996.

Mazarakis, Nicholas. “fightsma.” EIAV Viral Vectors in Gene Therapy of Spinal Muscular Atrophy fightsma 2003. Jan. 2005 <www.fightsma.com>.

MDA Publications. Renewing Muscles and Nerves: Could Stem Cells Be the Ultimate Body Repair Kit? Quest Vol. 7 Apr. 2000.

Muscular Dystrophy Association: MDA Chat. Spinal Muscular Atrophy Research Update. MDAchat Nov. 2003 <www.azstarnet.com>.

Medline Plus. Hydroxurea. Medline Plus 2006. Aug. 2006 www.nlm.nih.gov/medlineplus/>.

Medline Plus. Sodium Phenylbutyrate. Medline Plus Jan. 2006 <www.nlm.nig.gov>.

Monani, Umrao R. Neuron “A Deficiency in Ubiquitous Protein: A Motor Neuron Specific Disease” Vol. 48, Dec. 2005. Feb. 2006.

Motor Neuron Disease Association. Stem Cells and Motor Neuron Disease June 2005.

MrSci.com. Neurons. MrSci.com Jan. 2006 <www.mrsci.com/Neuroscience>.

Musat, Theodore. “Spinal Muscular Atrophy.” The Spinal Muscular Atrophies/ MDA Research Jan. 2006. MDA 24 Aug 2006 <www.mdausa.org>.

National Institute of Neurological Disorders and Stroke. NINDS Motor Neuron Diseases Information Page. NINDS Jan. 2006 <www.ninds.nih.gov>.

National Institute of Neurological Disorders and Stroke. Valproic Acid Shows Promise for Treating Spinal Muscular Atrophy. NINDS Jan. 2006.

National Institutes of Health. Stem Cells and Diseases: The Promise of Stem Cells NIH 2006 <www.stemcells.nih.gov>.

National Institutes of Health. Stem Cell Information: Executive Summary NIH Aug. 2005 <www.stemcells.nih.gov>.

National Institutes of Health. Rebuilding the Nervous System with Stem Cells Stem Cell Information 2006 <www.stemcells.nih.gov/>.

National Institutes of Health. Use of Genetically Modified Stem Cells in Experimental Gene Therapies Stem Cell Information 2006 <www.stemcells.nih.gov/>.

National Institutes of Health. Autoimmune Diseases and the Promise of Stem Cell-Based Therapies Stem Cell Information 2006 <www.stemcells.nih.gov>.

NCBI PubMed. Distinct and Overlapping Alterations in Motor and Sensory Neurons in a Mouse Model of Spinal Muscular Atrophy. PubMed Jan. 2006 <www.ncbi.nlm.nih.gov >.

NCBI PubMed. Pilot Trial of Phenylbutyrate in Spinal Muscular Atrophy. PubMed Feb. 2004 <www.ncbi.nlm.nih.gov>.

NCBI Pub/Med. Intravenous Administration of Human Umbilical Cord Blood Cells in a Mouse Model of Amyotrophic Lateral Sclerosis: Distribution, Migration, and Differentiation PubMed Abstract Jun. 2003 <www.ncbi.nlm.nih.gov>.

Oxford BioMedica. Oxford Biomedica Publishes Preclinical Efficacy Results with Its Product Candidate SMN1-G For Spinal Muscular Atrophy. Oxford Biomedica Dec. 2006.

Perlman, Spencer. "Newborn Screening Saves Lives Act Introduced in the U.S. Senate." Families of Spinal Muscular Atrophy 16(2006):4-5.

Peterson, Cynthia M. "Stem Cell Research." Women for Faith and Family Oct. 2004. Jan. 2006 <www.wff.org>.

Robertson, George S. et al. "Blackwell Synergy" Neuroprotection by the Inhibition of Apoptosis. Brain Pathology, Abstract Apr. 2000 <www.blackwell-synergy.com>.

Schmeck, Harold. "Howard Hughes Medical Institution." Why So Many Errors in Our DNA Blazing a Genetic Trail 2006. Jul. 2006 <www.hhmi.org>.

SCID Homepage. Missing Body Defense Systems 2004. Jul. 2006 <www.scid.net>.

Science and Theology News. An Alternate Use for PGD Science and Theology News 2006 <www.religioustolerance.org>.

Sejong, Shin et al. "American Chemical Society." An Anti-Apoptotic Protein Human Survivin Is a Direct Inhibitor of Caspae-3 and-7" Jul. 2001 <www.pubs.acs.org>.

Simons, M. et al. "Blackwell Synergy." Adenovirus-Mediated Gene Transfer of Apoptosis Proteins Delays Apoptosis in Cerebellar Granule Neurons. Journal of Neurochemistry Abstract Jan. 1999. Jul. 2006 <www.blackwell-synergy.com>.

SMA Foundation. A Review of Spinal Muscular Atrophy Literature. SMA Foundation Jan. 2005 <www.smafoundation.org>.

Snyder, Dr. Evan and Lieberman, Bruce. "SignonSanDiego." Researchers Are in the Biology 101 Stage of Learning the Potentials for Cures. The Promise of Stem Cells Dec. 2004 <www.signonsandiego.com/news>.

The Stop ALD Foundation. Stem Cell Transplants: An Explanation of Bone Marrow Transplants (BMTs) and Umbilical Cord Blood Transplants (UCBTs). Current Therapies Winter 2004/2005 <www.stopald.org>.

Swoboda, Kathryn J. et al. "Annals of Neurology." Natural History of Denervation in SMA: Relation to Age, SMN2 Copy Number, and Function 57 (2005).

Tagliaferro, Linda. The Complete Idiot's Guide to Decoding Your Genes. Indianapolis: Pearson Education Association 1999.

University of Leicester Biochemistry Department. Oligos 2006. Jan. 2006.

VA Research and Development. The Use of the Histone Deacetylase Inhibitor, Sodium Butyrate, to Promote Neuroprotection, Improve Motor Performance and Reduce Weight Loss in Huntington's Disease. VA Research and Development Oct. 2005 <:www.vard.com>.

Weiss, Rick. "Stem Cell Advance Reported" 23 Aug 2006:1.

Wikipedia. Alpha Motor Neuron Wikipedia Jul. 2006 <www.en.wikipedia.org>.

Wikipedia. Glutamic Acid Wikipedia Jul 2006 <www.en.wikipedia.org>.

Wikipedia. Histone Wikipedia Jul. 2006 <www.en.wikipedia.org>.

Wikipedia. Valproic acid Wikipedia Aug. 2006 <www.en.wikipedia.org>.

Wikipedia. Gene Therapy Wikipedia Aug. 2006 <www.en.wikipedia.org>.

Wikipedia. Virus Wikipedia Aug. 2006 <www.en.wikipedia.org>.

Wikipedia. Gene Therapy Wikipedia Aug. 2006 <www.en.wikipedia.org>.

Wikipedia. Adrenoleukodystrophy Wikipedia 2006 <www.en.wikipedia.org>.

Wikipedia. Oligonucleotide Wikipedia Aug. 2006 <www.en.wikipedia.org>.

Endnotes

[1] Musat, Theodore. "Spinal Muscular Atrophy." *The Spinal Muscular Atrophies/ MDA Research* Jan. 2006. MDA 24 Aug 2006 <www.mdausa.org>. Type I SMA is the most common cause of genetically determined neonatal death with an incidence of 1 in 25,708 or 5-7 per 100,000. Herrera-Sot, Jose. Spinal Muscular Atrophy. emedicine. Oct. 2004. Jan. 2006 <www.emedicine.com>. It is the third most common diagnosis of neuromuscular disease seen in clinics for children under 18. Hirtz, D. *Challenges and Opportunities in Clinical Trials for Spinal Muscular Atrophy.* Neurology. 2005. 2006 <www.neurology.com>. One in every forty to fifty people is a carrier. The disease may have originated in Saudi Arabia where the incidence of SMA is considerably higher, most likely as the result of consanguinity (similar blood types).

[2] ... or noncarriers as the case may be. In most cases, each parent is lacking in one gene called the Survival of Motor Neuron (SMN) I gene. Typically, the child is deleted for this gene from both the mother and the father. However, there is a back-up SMN II gene (found only in humans) that minimally compensates for the SMN I gene. Thus, SMA is caused by the existence of SMN II gene as the SMN II gene can only produce enough SMN protein to sustain a fetus or newborn.

[3] Musat, Theodore. "Spinal Muscular Atrophy." *The Spinal Muscular Atrophies/ MDA Research* Jan. 2006. MDA 24 Aug 2006 <www.mdausa.org>.

Type I (severe) symptoms = 0-6 mos.; course = never sits; death = <2 yrs
Type II (intermediate) symptoms = 7-18 mos.; course = never stands; death = >2 yrs
Type III (mild) symptoms = >18 mos.; course = stands alone; death = adult

[4] Musat, Theodore. "Spinal Muscular Atrophy." *The Spinal Muscular Atrophies/ MDA Research* Jan. 2006. MDA 24 Aug 2006 <www.mdausa.org>. It is unknown whether the motor neurons are dying, in atrophy, or have not matured. This is a vitally important distinction in order to properly pursue a treatment or cure. See: SMA Foundation, *A Review of Spinal Muscular Atrophy Literature.* SMA Foundation. Jan. 2005. Jan. 2006 <www.smafoundation.org>.

[5] Musat, Theodore. “Spinal Muscular Atrophy.” *The Spinal Muscular Atrophies/MDA Research* Jan. 2006. MDA 24 Aug 2006 <www.mdausa.org>. A proximal weakness affectation means that the disease attacks muscles closest to the central body. For example, shoulders are weaker than the forearms, which are weaker than the hands, which are weaker than the fingers. Weakness in the legs is also characteristically greater in the legs than in the arms. Hypotonia is a lack of muscle tone.

[6] Dr. John R. Bach devised a protocol that does not necessitate tracheotomy. Rather, the patient uses a machine similar to one that people with sleep apnea use called a Bi Pap (Bi level Intermittent Positive air pressure). The protocol also includes frequent chest physical therapy along with vibration and a cough machine to clear the lungs from mucous build-up. Bach, John R. *Management of Patients with Neuromuscular Disease.* Philadelphia: Hanley & Belfus, Inc. 2004.

[7] www.smasupport.org

[8] Musat, Theodore. “Spinal Muscular Atrophy.” *The Spinal Muscular Atrophies/MDA Research* Jan. 2006. MDA 24 Aug 2006 <www.mdausa.org>. Weakness in muscles surrounding the diaphragm cause paradoxical or belly breathing. Illness occurs due to inability to clear lungs of mucous resulting in pneumonia. The affected person cannot cough or sneeze and has little or no gag reflex. Respiratory insufficiency, difficulty sucking and swallowing, accumulation of secretions and a weak cry are also characteristic of the disease. See also: Hirtz, D. *Challenges and Opportunities in Clinical Trials for Spinal Muscular Atrophy.* Neurology. 2005. 2006 <www.neurology.com>.

[9] “Fight SMA: Fact Sheet.” *FightSMA: Accelerating a Cure for Spinal Muscular Atrophy.* Aug. 2006. 24 Aug. 2006 <www.fightsma.com> Wolf Blitzer asked in a June 10, 2003 interview on CNN with “Fight SMA” former spokesperson Howie Long: “What is spinal muscular atrophy and why haven’t we heard more about it?” Anecdotally, few people with whom I have discussed my daughter’s condition or my niece’s death have ever heard of the disease. Most families affected by the disease will confirm this experience.

[10] Musat, Theodore. “Spinal Muscular Atrophy.” *The Spinal Muscular Atrophies/MDA Research* Jan. 2006. MDA 24 Aug 2006 <www.mdausa.org>. While SMA is considered by most to be a progressive disease, there is no objective evidence of this, and experienced clinicians suggest otherwise. It is more likely that the

observed functional deterioration in patients and resulting death leaves little opportunity to determine progression, whereas in types II and III the change is slow and difficult to measure.

[11] Musat, Theodore. "Spinal Muscular Atrophy." *The Spinal Muscular Atrophies/ MDA Research* Jan. 2006. MDA 24 Aug 2006 <www.mdausa.org>. SMA has been chosen by the National Institute of Health to be a model for translational research because it is the closest to a treatment out of 300 neurological diseases. See also: "Fight SMA: Fact Sheet." *FightSMA: Accelerating a Cure for Spinal Muscular Atrophy.* Aug. 2006. 24 Aug. 2006 <www.fightsma.com>.

[12] Schmeck, Harold. "Howard Hughes Medical Institution." *Why So Many Errors in Our DNA.* Blazing a Genetic Trail 2006. Jul. 2006 <www.hhmi.org/ genetictrail/d120.html> Much of DNA is riddled with errors; most are harmless. Considering the tremendous difficulties involved in protein transcription from DNA, it is a miracle that life exists at all. For example, every cell in the human body contains six feet of DNA, and every human cell consists of six billion subunits, or base pairs, coiled and tightly packed into twenty-three pairs of chromosomes, all of which must be duplicated every time a cell divides. Bits of DNA may be deleted, inserted, broken, or substituted. To stay alive and functioning, the human body requires a daily crop of billions of fresh protein molecules: about 40,000 different kinds of proteins that must be supplied in the right quantities, at the right times, and in the right places. Problems arise only when an error in DNA alters a message that tells certain cells to manufacture a certain protein, such as the SMN protein.

[13] Schmeck, Harold. "Howard Hughes Medical Institution." *Why So Many Errors in Our DNA.* Blazing a Genetic Trail 2006. Jul. 2006 <www.hhmi.org/ genetictrail/d120.html> This strategy has led to spectacular progress toward preventing or treating cystic fibrosis, Duchenne muscular dystrophy, neurofibromatosis, and other inherited disorders.

[14] HDAC Inhibitors are a class of drugs that upregulate the SMN protein necessary for motor neuron growth and function. See footnote 36 for further definition and description.

[15] Gene therapy is a form of therapy that can repair or replace a faulty or deleted gene through the introduction of a new gene with the use of a virus. See footnote 59 for further definition and description.

[16] Stanford University: Dr. Wang SMA I, Hydroxyurea; Utah: Dr. Swoboda, SMA II Carnitine and Valproic Acid; upcoming PNCR Network for SMA North-Eastern Clinical Trials Consortium: Columbia-Harvard-U. of Pennsylvania: SMA I Phase I clinical trial of Sodium Phenylbutyrate.

[17] Leading researcher Dr. Darryl DeVivo of Columbia University states that the optimal time to treat the disease is before SMA patients show clinical signs of it (that is, during the subacute phase). This means that treatment should begin before the underlying defects have initiated. In the most severe SMA cases (SMA I), this pre-clinical window would likely only be detected by prenatal screening for SMA. "fightsma." *Research News* 2004. Jul. 2005 <www.fightsma.com>. Arthur Burghes of Ohio State University has performed mouse studies that suggest that SMN may be required very early in development and that even high levels of SMN, if delivered too late, are not sufficient to prevent SMA development. "fightsma." *Research News.* 2004 Jul. 2005 <www.fightsma.com>.

[18] See footnote 73 for additional information.

[19] Perlman, Spencer. "Newborn Screening Saves Lives Act Introduced in the U.S. Senate." *Families of Spinal Muscular Atrophy* 16(2006): 4-5. Research indicates that for maximum effectiveness, SMA therapies will need to be given prior to significant motor neuron degeneration, which occurs during the pre-symptomatic phase in Type I. Also see footnote 15.

[20] In the spring of 2005, the Congressional Advisory Committee on Heritable Disorders released an initial uniform newborn panel comprised of 29 diseases and disorders for which it encourages states to screen newborns. Shockingly, SMA was not included in this list, nor was it among the original list of 84 diseases and disorders considered for inclusion in the list. Perlman, Spencer. "Newborn Screening Saves Lives Act Introduced in the U.S. Senate." *Families of Spinal Muscular Atrophy* 16(2006): 4-5.

[21] "Cell Suicide in Health and Disease". *Scientific American* Dec. 1996. Jul. 2006 <www.critpath.org/aric/library/art006.htm>. Evidence suggests that SMN protein plays a crucial role as a neuronal apoptotic inhibitor protein ("NAIP"). Cells can and often do kill themselves in a process known as apoptosis. This capacity is essential to the proper functioning of the body. For example, cells that become infected by a virus or that sustain irreparable genetic mutations often commit suicide (for the good of the whole body, organ or tissue). The failure of a genetically

altered cell to commit suicide can contribute to the development of cancer. Apoptosis may be set in motion by various triggers, including withdrawal from a cell of the chemical signals (known as growth, or survival, factors) through which cells reassure one another of their importance. Death also can be triggered by a cell's receipt of external or internal messages that override the reassuring ones or by the cell's receipt of conflicting directives as to whether it should divide. Apoptosis is regulated by the protein Bcl-2 and its family of related molecules (with such names as Bax and Bad). Some of these molecules block apoptosis while others promote it. Examples of apoptosis include: (1) development of the eye lens that forms during embryonic development. (consisting of apoptotic cells that have replaced their innards with clear protein cystallin); (2) skin cells, which begin life in the deepest layers and then migrate to the surface in layers, undergoing apoptosis along the way (and causing the resulting dead layer to form the protective outer skin layer, called the epidermis); and (3) the cells of the uterine wall, which die and are sloughed off during menstruation (accomplished by apoptosis).

[22] The gene used for gene therapy is formed from stem cells.

[23] Many types of motor neurons exist, and they differ in appearance. Characteristically, neurons are highly asymmetric in shape and consist of:

(1) the dendrite, a short branching arbor of cellular extensions. Each neuron has many dendrites. These structures form the main receiving network for the neuron.

(2) the soma, or cell-body, the relatively large central part of the cell between the dendrites and the axon.

(3) the axon, a much finer cable-like projection that may extend tens, hundreds, or even tens of thousands of times the diameter of the soma. Many neurons have insulating sheaths of myelin around their axons. The sheaths enable faster transmission signals and prevent short circuits among intersecting neurons. Neurons communicate with one another and to other cells through synapses, where the axon tip of one cell impinges upon a dendrite or soma of another. MrSci.com, *Neurons.* MrSci.com Jan. 2006 <www.mrsci.com/Neuroscience/Neuron.php> Upon stimulation, the motor neuron releases a flood of neurotransmitters that bind to postsynaptic receptors and triggers a response in the muscle fiber. Motor Neuron anatomy and physiology. Wikipedia, *Alpha Motor Neuron.* Wikipedia Jun. 2006. Jul. 2006 <www.wikipedia.org/wiki/Alpha motor neuron>

[24] In SMA I, clinical symptoms become apparent early but appear to stabilize over time. The phenomenon of preservation of strength in the setting of loss of function is well documented scientifically and anecdotally. Reinnervation of muscle fibers by the remaining motor neurons concurrent with progressive motor neuron loss would allow for prolonged periods of strength despite disease progression. Swoboda, Kathryn J. et al. "Annals of Neurology." *Natural History of Denervation in SMA: Relation to Age, SMN2 Copy Number, and Function* 57 (2005). This is particularly interesting for potential motor neuron therapy, because it demonstrates that compensation does occur and perhaps could be boosted or create a staging ground for axonal regrowth.

[25] National Institute of Neurological Disorders and Stroke, *NINDS Motor Neuron Diseases Information Page.* NINDS Jan. 2006. Feb. 2006 <www.ninds.nih.gov/disorders>

[26] NCBI PubMed, *Distinct and Overlapping Alterations in Motor and Sensory Neurons in a Mouse Model of Spinal Muscular Atrophy.* PubMed Jan. 2006. Feb. 2006 <www.ncbi.nlm.nih.gov/entrez>

[27] SMA Foundation, *A review of Spinal Muscular Atrophy Literature.* SMA Foundation. Jan. 2005. Jan. 2006 <www.smafoundation.org>. The protein processes molecules called messenger RNA ("mRNA") that serve as genetic blueprints for making other proteins. The transition from gene to protein is highly complex. There are two major steps: transcription and translation. During the process of transcription, the information stored in a gene's DNA is transferred to a similar molecule called RNA (ribonucleic acid) in the cell nucleus. Messenger RNA (mRNA) carries the "recipe" for the necessary protein from the DNA in the nucleus to the outer portion of the cell called the cytoplasm where the protein factories (ribosomes) make the necessary protein; this process is "translation". Tagliaferro, Linda. *The Complete Idiot's Guide to Decoding Your Genes.* Indianapolis: Pearson Education Association, 1999. Before the information can be brought to the factory, it must be transcribed from the DNA. This is called pre-mRNA. For example, when taking notes from a book, we copy only the most important information and cut out the unimportant material. This is how the pre-mRNA process works. Once edited, the mRNA is ready for processing. To put it another way, instructions in a gene need to be "read" when a cell needs to make a particular protein. DNA that makes up the gene unwinds and the message (into pre-mRNA) that is transcribed into another chemical called mRNA. This chemical takes the coded genetic information to the ribosome where it is

translated into a chain of amino acids that comprise the protein. The SMN protein is made up of 294 amino acids. Center for Genetics Education, *Genes and Chromosomes.* Center for Genetics Education 2006. Jul. 2006 <www.genetics.com> Many disease-associated mutations affect pre-mRNA splicing that cause inappropriate exonic skipping. Cartegni, Krainer. "NCBI PubMed" *Correction of Disease-Associated Exon Skipping by Synthetic Exon-Specific Activators.* NCBI PubMed Abstract Feb. 2003. Jul. 2006 <www.ncbi.nlm.nih.gov/entrez>

[28] Genetics Home Reference, *SMN1.* Genetics Home Reference Jul. 2006. Jul. 2006 <www.ghr.nlm.nih.gov/gene=smn1>. Interestingly, SMN levels are highest during embryonic development and drop postnatally by day seven. It is likely that this period defines when a minimum level of SMN must be maintained to ensure the health (for normal development) of motor neurons. Monani, Umrao R. *Neuron* "A Deficiency in Ubiquitous Protein; A Motor Neuron Specific Disease." Vol. 48, Dec. 2005. Feb. 2006. Also see: Dreyfus, Gideon. "Howard Hughes Medical Institute" *Ribonucleoprotein Complexes:Assembly, Function, and Roles in Human Disease.* HHMI Jan. 2006. Jul 2006 <www.hhmi.org/>.

[29] The Sahn Laboratory at Children's Hospital Boston hypothesizes that SMN may play a role in transport and/or translational regulation of RNAs necessary for axon growth and/or guidance of motor neurons. Thus, if SMN is missing, the axons cannot connect with their target muscles, leading to spinal motor neuron death and weakness. Darras, Dr. "Scientific Research Update." *From the Desk of Dr. Darras.* Aug. 2006.

[30] Jones, Kevin et al. "JBC Online" *Direct Interaction of the Spinal Muscular Atrophy Disease Protein SMN with the Small Nucleolar RNA-Associated Protein Fibrillarin.* JBC Online Abstract Aug. 2001. Jul. 2006 <www.jbc.org>. The health of all multicellular organisms depends on the body's ability to produce new cells and of individual cells to self-destruct when they become unnecessary, disordered, or dangerous to tissue, organ or body. The process of cell suicide is called apoptosis. Aberrant regulation of apoptosis (too much or too little) can cause cancer, AIDS, Alzheimer's, arthritis and other diseases. Critpath.org, *Cell Suicide in Health and Disease.* Scientific American Dec. 1996. Jul. 2006 <www.critpath.org/aric/library/art006.htm>. Inappropriate initiation or inhibition of apoptosis could contribute to SMA. Neuronal apoptotic inhibitors would downregulate apoptotic processes within the motor neurons. Without neuronal apoptotic inhibitors, apoptosis may run rampant and destroy motor neurons.

[31] Buss, Robert R. et al. *Annual Reviews.* "Adaptive Roles of Programmed Cell Death During Nervous System Development". Mar. 2006. Jul. 2006 < arjournals.annualreviews.org>

[32] Buss, Robert R. et al. *Annual Reviews.* "Adaptive Roles of Programmed Cell Death During Nervous System Development". Mar. 2006. Jul. 2006.

[33] Buss, Robert R. et al. *Annual Reviews.* "Adaptive Roles of Programmed Cell Death During Nervous System Development". Mar. 2006. Jul. 2006. Overexpression of neurotrophic (nourishing) factors can reduce neuronal cell death in some populations, which suggests that neurons may normally die through a lack of these factors. Lindsay, RM. "NCBI PubMed" *Trophic Protection of Motor Neurons: Clinical Potential in Motor Neuron Diseases.* NCBI PubMed Abstract Dec. 1994. Feb. 2006 <www.ncbi.nlm.nih.gov/entrez> See also: Jablonka, Sibylle. "Wiley Interscience" *Axonal Defects in Mouse Models of Motoneuron Disease.* Wiley Interscience Abstract Dec. 2003. Jul. 2006 <www3. interscience.wiley.com>. Cell death may also result from accumulation of excitatory amino acids, such as the neurotransmitter glutamate. Glutamate is a key molecule in cellular metabolism. In humans, dietary proteins are broken down by digestion into amino acids, which serves as metabolic fuel or other functional roles in the body. In excess, glutamic acid triggers a process called excitotoxicity causing neuronal damage and eventual cell death. Wikipedia, *Glutamic Acid.* 2006. Jul 2006 <www.en.wikipedia.org/wiki/glutamate>.

[34] Cell death might be limited by drugs that block free radical production or inhibit ice-like proteases (central cell executioners). Critpath.org, *Cell Suicide in Health and Disease.* Scientific American Dec. 1996. Jul. 2006 <www.critpath.org/aric/library/art006.htm>. Activation of cysteine protease caspase 3 appears to be a key event in execution of apoptosis in the central nervous system. Caspase 3 activation has been observed in stroke and spinal cord trauma. Peptide-based caspase inhibitors prevent neuronal loss in animal models. Robertson, George S. et al. "Blackwell Synergy" *Neuroprotection by the Inhibition of Apoptosis.* Brain Pathology, Abstract Apr. 2000. Jul. 2006 <www.blackwell-synergy.com/doi/abs/10.1111/j.1750-3639.2000.tb00262.x>. Inhibition of caspases delays but does not prevent cell death. Thus, continued slow death without caspase activation may be associated with DNA fragmentation. Although dysregulation of apoptosis can result in inappropriate suppression of cell death (that could lead to cancer or tumor growth), failure to initially control the extent of cell death may be even more dangerous: SMA I is more often than not a death sentence. Liston, P. et al.

"NCBI PubMed" *Suppression of Apoptosis in Mammalian Cells by NAIP and a Related Family of IAP Genes.* Nature abstract Jan. 1996. Jul. 2006 <www.ncbi.nlm.nih.gov/entrez>.

[35] Sejong, Shin et al. "American Chemical Society." *An Anti-Apoptotic Protein Human Survivin Is A Direct Inhibitor of Caspae-3 and-7* Jul. 2001. Jul. 2006 <www.pubs.acs.org>. Whether survivin is a physiologically relevant caspase inhibitor has been unclear due to the difficulties of obtaining correctly folded survivin and finding the right conditions for inhibition assay.

[36] See footnote 34.

[37] Katsuno, Masahisa et al. "ScienceDirect." *Testosterone Reduction Prevents Phenotypic Expression in a Transgenic Mouse Model of Spinal and Bulbar Muscular Atrophy* Neuron (35) Aug. 2002. Aug. 2006 <www.sciencedirect.com/science?_ob=ArticleURL&-udi=B6WSS-4CC2Y9F-43&_coverDa …>. For example, testosterone reduction has been shown to prevent phenotypic expression of SMA in a mouse model of SMA. Thus, hormonal intervention to diminish testosterone level can be applied to human therapy. While it may not entirely halt the progression, it may be able to slow it down enough to begin an effective regimen of upregulation of SMN protein. The HDAC Inhibitor Sodium Phenylbutyrate may also act as an anti-apoptotic agent.

[38] Binhai Zheng. "Roman Reed Program Research Grants." *Functional Analysis of Nogo in CNS Axon Regeneration Using a Nogo Null Mutant.* RRPRG 2005. Feb. 2006 <www.reeve.uci.edu/romanreed/grants2004.php>.

[39] This protein stops axons from regrowing after injury. The Nogo protein is like a key that fits into a lock, called a receptor, which is located on an axon. Turning the receptor lock with the Nogo key stops regeneration. Preventing Nogo's action can potentially be accomplished in two ways: (1) change the shape of the Nogo protein so that it no longer fits in the receptor, or (2) jam or change the lock. Cocco, Melanie. "Roman Reed Program Research Grants." *Structure of Proteins That Inhibit CNS Repair: Nogo and its Receptor.* RRPRG 2005. Feb. 2006 <www.reeve.uci.edu/romanreed/grants2005.php>.

[40] Binhai Zheng. "Roman Reed Program Research Grants." *Functional Analysis of Nogo in CNS Axon Regeneration Using a Nogo Null Mutant.* RRPRG 2005. Feb. 2006 <www.reeve.uci.edu/romanreed/grants2004.php>. None of these models completely disrupts or knocks out the Nogo gene. However, Dr. Zheng has

developed a model that completely eliminates Nogo. This model may allow him to fully characterize the role of Nogo in blocking regeneration. If his mice show good regeneration, this would provide strong evidence that regeneration can be enhanced with the removal of Nogo from the cellular environment.

[41] "Columbia University Medical Center: INVIVO." *Scientists Crack Neuron Code.* Jan. 2006. Feb. 2006. In a study published in the Nov. 4 issue of Cell, Dr. Jessel and postdoctoral researcher Jeremy Dasen describe that the allegiances are formed with a code based on 21 different Hox genes, which encode proteins that regulate gene expression.

Theoretically, turning off Nogo while simultaneously turning on Hox genes may stimulate regeneration.

[43] "Columbia University Medical Center: INVIVO." *Scientists Crack Neuron Code.* Jan. 2006. Feb. 2006.

[44] The SMN2 gene does not produce enough full-length protein because, during transcription, an important segment of RNA known as an exon is omitted. Exons are important pieces of the "recipe" for the protein along the DNA strand that are broken up by introns, which are blank spaces between the exons. Exon 7 deletion results in a truncated and highly unstable SMN protein. Only about ten percent of its protein is useful, full-length protein. Hertel, Klemens. Abstract: "Correction of SMN2 Pre-mRNA Splicing by Antisense U7 Small Nuclear RNAs" *Families of Spinal Muscular Atrophy* 15 (2006):1. Full-length SMN appears to interact with two binding proteins that will not interact with the truncated SMN protein. This two-protein complex appears to modulate (and is therefore necessary for) axonal growth. "Oxford BioMedica" Oxford Biomedica Publishes Preclinical Efficacy Results with it Product Candidate SMN1-G For Spinal Muscular Atrophy. *Oxford Biomedica* Dec. 2006. Jul. 2006 <www.oxfordbiomedica.co.uk/> This may contribute to the apparent confusion as to whether the motor neurons are dead or simply immature.

[45] The SMN1 gene produces full-length, stable SMN protein that acts as an anti-apoptotic agent. Interestingly, evidence suggests that the SMN2 gene product of truncated SMN protein may be converted from an anti-apoptotic agent to pro-apoptotic by skipping exon 7. Thus, mutant (lacking exon 7) SMN protein produced by the SMN2 gene may function as a regulator of the full-length SMN anti-apoptotic function (inhibitor of anti-apoptosis function). Kerr, Douglas A.

et al …" Proceedings of the National Academy of Sciences of the United States of America." abstract; Survival Motor Neuron Protein Modulates Neuron-Specific Apoptosis. *PNAS* Nov. 2000. Jul. 2006 <www.pnas.org>.

[46] Hertel, Klemens. Abstract: "Correction of SMN2 Pre-mRNA Splicing by Antisense U7 Small Nuclear RNAs" *Families of Spinal Muscular Atrophy* 15 (2006):1. As the baby grows, the amount of SMN protein remains constant, thereby causing the death of motor neurons. This is the genesis of the debate regarding the degree to which SMA I is progressive. There is little to no evidence that the disease is progressive. The primary contributing factor to this misnomer is simply the fact that the victims die so quickly. Musat, Theodore. "Spinal Muscular Atrophy." The Spinal Muscular Atrophies/MDA Research Jan. 2006. MDA 24 Aug 2006 <www.mdausa.org>. Once ninety percent of the motor neurons have died or atrophied, the disease does not progress. Anecdotally, children that survive the first two years appear to strengthen.

[47] For example, SMA I patients have one SMN2 gene thus producing only about ten percent of the necessary protein. They have a life expectancy of less than two years. SMA II patients may have two SMN2 genes producing twenty percent of full-length SMN protein. SMA II, while still deadly, has a slower progression; life expectancy is usually ten to fifteen years. Musat, Theodore. "Spinal Muscular Atrophy." The Spinal Muscular Atrophies/MDA Research Jan. 2006. MDA 24 Aug 2006 <www.mdausa.org>.

[48] In fact, even a slight percentage boost in neuronal function may be enough to transform a type I phenotype to that of a type II.

[49] Histones act as spools around which the DNA winds; they play a role in gene regulation and expression. For example, genes that are active (acetylated) have less bound (loose) histones and greater expression (more protein output). Tighter (deactylated) histones provide for less DNA expression. Histone deacetylation increases the histones' affinity for DNA (tightening the spool), thus down-regulating DNA (suppressing) transcription by blocking access to transcription factors. Deactylation inhibitors induce gene expression (loosening the spool), thus blocking deacetylation and increasing protein production. "Wikipedia." Histone. Wikipedia 2006. Jul. 2006 <www.en.wikipedia.org/wiki/Histone>. HDAC inhibitors boost SMN2 gene expression to produce more SMN protein by inhibiting deacetylation (loosening the spool). The hope is to boost the amount of full length SMN protein which, without the inhibitors, would remain at about ten

percent. Researchers theorize that boosting full-length SMN protein beyond ten percent would result in reduction of phenotype (greater motor neuron strength). "Wikipedia." Histone. Wikipedia 2006. Jul. 2006 <www.en.wikipedia.org/wiki/Histone>.

[50] "Medline Plus." Hydroxurea. Medline Plus 2006. Aug. 2006 <www.nlm.nih.gov/medlineplus/drugsinfo/uspki/202291.html>.

[51] Hydroxyurea interferes with the growth of cancer cells. "Medline Plus." Hydroxurea. Medline Plus 2006. Aug. 2006 <www.nlm.gov/medlineplus/drugsinfo/uspki/202291.html>. Specifically, hydroxyurea is used in hematological malignancies such as chronic myeloggenous leukemia. It is also used for treatment of sickle cell anemia, thalassemia, and AIDS. Side effects include drowsiness, nausea, vomiting, diarrhea, constipation, hair loss, anemia, and abnormal liver enzymes. Close monitoring through blood testing is strongly recommended. "Wikipedia." Histone. Wikipedia 2006. Jul. 2006 <www.en.wikipedia.org/wiki/Histone>.

[52] The tests were performed on cultured cells from patients with SMA and in time-related and dose dependent increases in the ratio of full-length to truncated SMN messenger RNA. SMN protein levels and "gems" also were significantly increased in the hydroxyurea-treated cells. Grzeschik, Susanna M. et al. "Wiley Interscience." Hydroxyurea Enhances SMN2 Gene Expression in Spinal Muscular Atrophy Cells. Abstract *Wiley Interscience* Jul. 2005. Jul. 2006 <www3.interscience.wiley.com>.

[53] Conger, Krista. "Stanford School of Medicine" Drug Provides Glimmer of Hope for Children Suffering Fatal Genetic Disease. Stanford Oct. 2005. Aug. 2006 <www.med.stanford.edu>.

[54] "… I decided then that I had to do something about this … at that point we didn't have a clue about the pathogenesis of the disease," says Wang. "Kids just died." Wang advanced his ideas at an international SMA meeting in 1996 while other researchers were discussing how to use gene therapy to produce the full-length protein. "I stood up and said Look, we already have a copy of the gene there in the DNA. I think we can do something about this disease if we can make this spare copy work like the real one.… They all just looked at me thoughtfully." Conger, Krista. "Stanford School of Medicine" Denying Death: A Baby-Killing

Disease Meets its Match. Stanford Spring 2006. Aug. 2006 <www.mednews.stanford.edu>.

[55] "She [the patient] needed less help breathing and was less likely to choke." Conger, Krista. "Stanford School of Medicine" Denying Death: A Baby-Killing Disease Meets its Match. Stanford Spring 2006. Aug. 2006 <www.mednews.stanford.edu>.

[56] "… her left leg started to rotate, she was pushing with her feet … her arms became stronger … She also needed less help breathing and was less likely to choke." "Stanford School of Medicine" Denying Death: A Baby-Killing Disease Meets its Match. Stanford Spring. 2006. Aug. 2006 <www.mednews.stanford.edu/stanmed/2006spring/wang.html>. Even these gains can be linked to factors other than the drug. For example, if the patient lost weight during the trial, strength would appear to have gained due to noticeable increased movement. In fact, it may just be easier to move and breathe after even mere ounces of weight loss.

[57] Irwin, Joseph et al. "Families of Spinal Muscular Atrophy" abstract: SMA Research Update from the Families of SMA Supported Research Meeting. FSMA Aug. 2006. Aug. 2006 <www.curesma.org>. Dr. Wang reported that the safety profile is reasonable and a responder group with increased SMN levels was reported, "although it was unclear at this point whether these patients have received drug as they [sic] study is still blinded."

[58] Cassandra began hydroxyurea at the age of ten months. While on higher dosages of hydroxyurea than the Stanford study (8 ml/day at 38 pounds), she continued to lose motor function and deteriorated to the point of losing her smile and requiring a twenty-four hour Bi-Pap respirator.

[59] Our objective was for Cassandra to reduce body mass to the fiftieth percentile bracket.

[60] "Wikipedia." Valproic acid. Wikipedia Aug. 2006. Aug. 2006 <www.en.wikipedia.org>. The drug also is being studied for its effectiveness in the treatment of leukemia in juvenile patients.

[61] Common side effects are dyspepsia and/or weight gain. Less common are dysphoria, fatigue, dizziness, drowsiness, hair loss, headaches, nausea, sedation, and tremors. Rarely, valproic acid can cause dyscarsia, impaired liver function, jaun-

dice, and prolonged coagulation times. Consult with a doctor for other effects. Treatment with valproic acid can lead to liver toxicity especially in children under two. "National Institute of Neurological Disorders and Stroke." Valproic Acid Shows Promise for Treating Spinal Muscular Atrophy. NINDS Jan. 2006. Feb. 2006 <www.ninds.gov>.

[62] "National Institute of Neurological Disorders and Stroke." Valproic Acid Shows Promise for Treating Spinal Muscular Atrophy. NINDS Jan. 2006. Feb. 2006 <www.ninds.gov>.

[63] "BBC News." Self-Repair Gene Therapy Promise. BBC News May 2006. May 2006 <www.news.bbc.co.uk/2/hi/health/4976984/stm>. The team first treated ten parents of children with SMA with valproate for four months. However, researchers cautioned that yet unclear is whether SMN expression in blood reflects SMN expression in motor neurons and therefore has an effect on muscle strength. Further details of the study were given recently at the June 2006 FSMA Researchers Conference. The study showed that seven of ten carriers' mRNA levels increased. Three carriers did not show change. Irwin, Joseph et al. "Families of Spinal Muscular Atrophy" abstract: SMA Research Update from the Families of SMA Supported Research Meeting. FSMA Aug. 2006. Aug. 2006 <www.curesma.org/res2006news.shtml>.

[64] "National Institute of Neurological Disorders and Stroke." Valproic Acid Shows Promise for Treating Spinal Muscular Atrophy. NINDS Jan. 2006. Feb. 2006 <www.ninds.gov>.

[65] Another study in the use of valproic acid for the treatment of SMA at Washington University School of Medicine found similar positive results. However, the lead investigator, Dr. Chris Weihl (a postdoctoral fellow in neurology) acknowledges that valproate may not work as well in "those patients [younger SMA I]" but that they would make sure "researchers did not discard the possibility that valproate may help older sufferers even if the trials in pediatric patients went poorly." Acharya, Sanjukta. "RxPG News Muscular Dystrophies Channel." Valproate Effective in Adult Spinal Muscular Atrophy. RxPG News Jun. 2006. Jun. 2006 <www.rxpgnews.com>. In fact the clinical trial where these positive results were garnered excluded anyone under the age of seventeen, those with the mildest form of the disease. "CBC News." Valproate Helped People with SMA Get Stronger. CBC News Jun. 2006. Jul. 2006 <www.cbc.ca/cp/HealthScout/>.

The headline is again misleading in that there is a vast divide between the almost always lethal SMA I and the milder forms of strong SMA II and III.

[66] Ammonia is formed from the breakdown of protein in the body. If the body cannot remove ammonia, then a buildup may cause serious unwanted effects.

[67] This option is being pursued due to its inhibitory effects in cell proliferation models. "VA Research and Development." The Use of the Histone Deacetylase Inhibitor, Sodium Butyrate, to Promote Neuroprotection, Improve Motor Performance and Reduce Weight Loss in Huntington's Disease. VA Research and Development Oct. 2005. Feb. 2006 <www.vard.org>.

[68] "VA Research and Development." The Use of the Histone Deacetylase Inhibitor, Sodium Butyrate, to Promote Neuroprotection, Improve Motor Performance and Reduce Weight Loss in Huntington's Disease. VA Research and Development Oct. 2005. Feb. 2006 <www.vard.org>. Also see: "NCBI PubMed." Pilot Trial of Phenylbutyrate in Spinal Muscular Atrophy. PubMed Feb. 2004. Feb. 2006 <www.ncbi.nlm.nih.gov/entrez>. The study was to evaluate tolerability and efficacy of SB.

[69] "NCBI PubMed." Pilot Trial of Phenylbutyrate in Spinal Muscular Atrophy. PubMed Feb. 2004. Feb. 2006 <www.ncbi.nlm.nih.gov>.

[70] No major side effects were noted in the study. "NCBI PubMed." Pilot Trial of Phenylbutyrate in Spinal Muscular Atrophy. PubMed Feb. 2004. Feb. 2006 <www.ncbi.nlm.nih.gov>. The study was to evaluate tolerability and efficacy of SB. However, some common side effects include change in frequency breathing, lack of or irregular mensturation, mood or mental changes, muscle pain or twitching, nausea or vomiting, nervousness or restlessness, lower back, side or stomach pain, swelling of feet or lower legs, unpleasant taste, and unusual tiredness or weakness. "Medline Plus." Sodium Phenylbutyrate. Medline Plus Jan. 2006. Feb. 2006 <www.nlm.nig.gov>.

[71] "Muscular Dystrophy Association: MDA Chat." Spinal Muscular Atrophy Research Update. MDAchat Nov. 2003. Feb. 2006 <http://database.azstarnet.com>.

[72] In fact, at the 2006 FSMA conference, Dr. Swoboda reported the results of a few individual patients who were younger than two. The hurdle was that it is quite difficult to administer the drug in adequate amounts (due to short half-life

in the body). Thus, alternatives are being investigated (in a new formulation) so that the medicine is easier to take. Irwin, Joseph et al. “Families of Spinal Muscular Atrophy” abstract: SMA Research Update from the Families of SMA Supported Research Meeting. FSMA Aug. 2006. Aug. 2006 <www.curesma.org>.

[73] “Wikipedia.” Gene Therapy 2006. Aug. 2006 <www.en.wikipedia.org/wiki/Gene_therapy>. Gene therapy is the insertion of genes into an individual’s cells and tissues to treat a disease (hereditary diseases in particular). Gene therapy aims to supplement a defective mutant allele with a functional one. Gene therapy began in the 1980s with scientists looking for a method of easily producing proteins, such as insulin that is deficient in diabetics. Scientists introduced human genes into bacterial DNA. The modified bacteria then produced the corresponding protein, which can be harvested and injected in people who cannot harvest it naturally.

[74] Mazarakis, Nicholas. “fightsma.” EIAV Viral Vectors in Gene Therapy of Spinal Muscular Atrophy fightsma 2003. Jan. 2005 <www.fightsma.com/rnews/mazarakis-art.asp>. Cells produce vital proteins from instructions they receive from the DNA located in the nucleus. DNA is copied “word- for- word” into RNA (a chemical cousin of DNA). The RNA is the template that cells use to make proteins. Prior to production of protein, the RNA is edited to remove excess “words” in a process called splicing. During the splicing of the defective SMN2 gene (SMN1 gene is deleted or non-functioning), an important segment of the RNA is left out (exon 7 is skipped resulting in the production of truncated SMN protein). A new “correct” gene would be introduced to produce full-length SMN protein.

[75] “Centre for Genetics Education.” Genes Therapy: Genes and Health Feb. 2004. Jul. 2006 <www.genetics.com/au/factsheet/25.htm>. See also: Mazarakis, Nicholas. “fightsma.” EIAV Viral Vectors in Gene Therapy of Spinal Muscular Atrophy fightsma 2003. Jan. 2005 <www.fightsma.com>.

[76] Mixed results of viral vector gene delivery systems have led researchers to seek alternative ways of delivering genes to the target host without the use of an inactivated virus. One of the most prominent methods has been the use of capsules to protect and guide the DNA into cells. Chemists have created virus-size structures to temporarily encase and protect genetic material, diffuse it through three-dimensional tissue, zero in on target cells, enter those cells and then release genetic cargoes at the proper location. Gorman, Jessica. “Science News.” Deliver-

ing the Goods: Gene Therapy Without the Virus Jan. 2003. Jul. 2006 <www.sciencenews.org>.

[77] Virus is Latin for poison. It is a submicroscopic particle that can infect cells of a biological organism. They are basic organisms that consist of genetic material contained within a protective protein shell. Viruses are intracellular parasites that lack the means of self-reproduction outside a host cell, but unlike parasites (which are living organisms), viruses are not considered to be alive because they do not meet all the criteria of the generally accepted definition of life (as do embryonic cells). In order to be considered "alive" an organism must possess a cell membrane or metabolize on its own. Viruses are also not made up of cells. The origins of viruses remain unclear. "Wikipedia." Virus 2006. Aug. 2006 <www.en.wikipedia.org>.

[78] "Wikipedia." Gene Therapy 2006. Aug. 2006 <www.en.wikipedia.org>. The virus has two genes, A and B. Gene A encodes a protein that allows this virus to insert itself into the host's genome. Gene B actually causes the disease with which the virus is associated. Scientists want to replace the B gene with a "good" or desirable gene. First a scientist would remove the genes in the virus that cause disease and replace them with genes that have the desired effect.

[79] Adenoviruses are viruses that carry their genetic material in the form of double-stranded DNA. They cause respiratory (e.g., common cold virus), intestinal, and eye infections. When these viruses attack a host cell, they introduce their DNA molecule into the host cell, and the instructions in this extra DNA molecule are transcribed just like any other gene. The only difference is that these extra genes are not replicated when the cell is about to undergo cell division. This type of virus would require re-administration in a growing cell population but could aid in the prevention of adverse effects such as cancer. In contrast, adeno-associated viruses have a single stranded form of DNA. This type of virus is being used because it is non-pathogenic (most people carry this harmless virus) and therefore does not trigger an immune response to newly treated cells. "Wikipedia." Gene Therapy 2006. Aug. 2006 <www.en.wikipedia.org>.

[80] Fear that alteration of genes would be passed to future generations was alleviated because only somatic cells are targeted for treatment. Thus, any changes to the genes of a person by gene therapy will only impact on the cells or their body and cannot be passed on to their children. That is because changes to the somatic cells cannot be inherited. Genetic alteration of sex cells (germ cells: sperm and

eggs) is still a controversial area within this field. "Centre for Genetics Education." Genes Therapy: Genes and Health Feb. 2004. Jul. 2006 <www.genetics.com.au>.

[81] "Wikipedia." Gene Therapy 2006. Aug. 2006 <www.en.wikipedia.org>.

[82] Dr. Anderson is a preeminent gene therapist at University of Southern California medical school.

[83] Dentzer, Susan. "Online NewsHour." Online Focus: Gene Therapy Dec. 1999. Jul. 2006 <www.pbs.org>. Severe combined immune deficiency (SCID) is the most severe of the primary immune deficiency diseases. It is also known as the "Bubble Boy" syndrome. In 1971, a boy was born with the disease (his older sibling had already died from the same disease) and immediately placed into a specially designed isolator crib where the air was specially filtered, and all items that went into the crib were sterilized. As he grew, so did his "bubble" area. At the age of twelve he walked out of his sterile environment and died shortly thereafter. The defining characteristic of SCID is the absence of T-cells. Unless this defect is corrected, the child will die of opportunistic infections before the first of second birthday. Like SMA, it is an autosomal recessive inheritance (meaning that the child inherits two defective copies of the same gene). "SCID Homepage." Missing Body Defense Systems 2004. Jul. 2006 <www.scid.net/about.htm>.

[84] They were T-cells carrying corrected DNA. Periodic tests on the patient showed that her re-engineered cells were not only surviving but producing the necessary ADA enzyme, proving that placement of a correct gene into a sufficient number of cells could correct the disease. Ashanti DeSilva remains healthy and vibrant. "SCID Homepage." Missing Body Defense Systems 2004. Jul. 2006 <www.scid.net/about.htm>.

[85] His was the first death directly attributed to the effects of the gene therapy rather than to the patient's underlying medical condition. A subsequent FDA investigation suggested that researchers at the university violated strict trial protocols. In fact, if the protocols had been followed, Gelsinger should never have been enrolled in the experiment. Because of a failure to get healthy copies of genes into enough cells of the body to reverse the underlying disease, researchers raised the dosage level of adenovirus vectors, running the risk of irritating his body's immune system. Seventeen patients had received the vector without problems, and Gelsinger was the eighteenth and last patient. Preliminary findings suggested

that Gelsinger had ammonia levels in his blood that were too high to participate in the trial. The high ammonia levels indicated that Gelsinger's liver function was working too poorly for him to be admitted into the study. Dentzer, Susan. "Online NewsHour." Online Focus: Gene Therapy Dec. 1999. Jul. 2006 <www.pbs.org>.

[86] Dentzer, Susan. "Online NewsHour." Online Focus: Gene Therapy Dec. 1999. Jul. 2006 <www.pbs.org>. In fact, patients with cystic fibrosis had such severe reactions to the therapy that trials were halted. Furthermore, efforts to treat patients with advanced heart disease, cancer, and AIDS did not stop progress of the underlying illness.

[87] The insertion of the corrected DNA into the defective cells had occurred next to a specific leukemia inhibitor. "SCID Homepage." Missing Body Defense Systems 2004. Jul. 2006 <www.scid.net/about.htm>.

[88] Currently, new SCID trials have begun or are in progress. It is still believed that gene therapy holds the greatest hope for a true cure for this disease. "SCID Homepage." Missing Body Defense Systems 2004. Jul. 2006 <www.scid.net/about.htm>.

[89] Fibroblasts are skin cells.

[90] In the nucleus of most cells SMN protein is concentrated in structures termed gems, which often co-localize with coiled bodies. In type I SMA patients, SMN levels are severely reduced and cells have few or no gems. Azzouz, Mimoun et al. "Lentivector-Mediated SMN Replacement in a Mouse Model of Spinal Muscular Atrophy" Journal of Clinical Investigation 114(2004): 1726.

[91] DiDonato, CJ et al. "NCBI/PubMed." abstract: Development of a Gene Therapy Strategy for the Restoration of Survival Motor Neuron Protein Expression: Implications for Spinal Muscular Atrophy PubMed Jan. 2003. Jul. 2006 <www.ncbi.nlm.nih.gov>. SMA Research Update from the Families of SMA Supported Research Meeting. FSMA Aug. 2006. Aug. 2006 <www.curesma.org>.

[92] Simons, M. et al. "Blackwell Synergy." Adenovirus-Mediated Gene Transfer of Apoptosis Proteins Delays Apoptosis in Cerebellar Granule Neurons, Journal of Neurochemistry Abstract Jan. 1999. Jul. 2006 <www.blackwell-synergy.com>.

[93] Oxford Biomedica is a leading gene therapy company. The company is working with Dr. Arthur Burghes of Ohio State University and is funded by Fight SMA. Most recently, it appears that progress has been stalled as Oxford BioMedica is seeking partners in the clinical development of the product. This may be due to the fact that it has such a comparatively low market value (approximately US $50 million). "Biomedica." Oxford Biomedica Publishes Preclinical Efficacy Results with its Product Candidate SMN1-G for Spinal Muscular Atrophy Oxford Biomedica Dec. 2004. Jul. 2006 <www.biomedica-usa.com>.

[94] Azzouz, Mimoun et al. "Lentivector-Mediated SMN Replacement in a Mouse Model of Spinal Muscular Atrophy" Journal of Clinical Investigation 114(2004): 1726. Their newly developed drug MoNuDin was underfunded by a US motor neuron charity and the ALS Association. The company is currently completing preclinical proof of principle studies, based on a study showing reduced levels of vascular endothelial growth factor (VEGF), by introducing the neuroprotective protein through its protein producing gene. In animal studies the therapy boosted survival rates by thirty percent. Market estimates for the drug are US $200 million. "Biomedica." MoNuDin: A Gene-Based Therapeutic for Motor Neuron Disease Product Profile Sep. 2005. Jul. 2006 <www.biomedica-usa.com>. See also: "Journal of Nature." May 2004 volume 429, Issue 6990, pp 413-417.

[95] Five SMA animals were injected with SMN-expressing lentivector. Five untreated animals were also included in the study. Analysis of the treated animals' body weight revealed delayed weight loss and delayed phenotypic presentation. They lost the ability to ambulate slightly later than those that were untreated. Their life span was extended by an average of three and five days compared to untreated animals. Untreated SMA mice develop phenotype five days after birth, first by a decrease in their body weight, followed by motor neuron loss starting at nine days of age. As the disease progresses, they also develop proximal muscle weakness and atrophy, resulting in end-stage paralysis and death at approximately 13.27 days of age. Azzouz, Mimoun et al. "Lentivector-Mediated SMN Replacement in a Mouse Model of Spinal Muscular Atrophy" Journal of Clinical Investigation 114(2004): 1726.

[96] Azzouz, Mimoun et al. "Lentivector-Mediated SMN Replacement in a Mouse Model of Spinal Muscular Atrophy" Journal of Clinical Investigation 114(2004): 1726.

[97] "National Institute of Health." Stem Cells and Diseases: The Promise of Stem Cells NIH 2006. Jul. 2006 <www.stemcells.nih.gov>.

[98] "National Institutes of Health." Stem Cell Information: Executive Summary NIH Aug. 2005. Jul. 2006 <www.stemcells.nih.gov>.

[99] "National Institute of Health." Stem Cells and Diseases: The Promise of Stem Cells NIH 2006. Jul. 2006 <www.stemcells.nih.gov>. A group led by Dr. James Thompson at the University of Wisconsin developed a technique to isolate and grow the cells. Limited federal funds to support hESC research have been available since August 9, 2001 when President Bush announced his decision on Federal funding for hESC research.

[100] "National Institutes of Health." Stem Cells and Diseases: The Promise of Stem Cells NIH 2006. Jul. 2006 <www.stemcells.nih.gov>. However, these newer uses have involved studies with a very limited number of patients.

[101] "National Institutes of Health." Stem Cell Information: Executive Summary NIH Aug. 2005. Jul. 2006 <www.stemcells.nih.gov>. More recently, scientists reported that adult stem cells from one tissue appear to be capable of developing into cells that are characteristic of other cells. Scientists also have discovered adult stem cells in tissues previously not thought to contain them, such as the brain.

[102] Hematopoietic stem cells (HSCs) are currently the only type of stem cells commonly used for therapy. "Cure Paralysis NOW Advocacy Group." What is an Embryonic Stem Cell (ESC)? Cure Paralysis Now May 2003. Jan. 2006 <www.cureparalysisnow.org>.

[103] "National Institutes of Health." Stem Cell Information: Executive Summary NIH Aug. 2005. Jul. 2006 <www.stemcells.nih.gov>. A new term arose to describe the ability of adult stem cells to differentiate into other types of cells and tissue: emerged-adult stem cell plasticity. The implication is that cells from the bone marrow (originally thought to be purely blood-forming cells) may contribute to regeneration of damaged livers, kidneys, hearts, lungs and other organs. "Cure Paralysis NOW Advocacy Group." What is an Embryonic Stem Cell (ESC)? Cure Paralysis Now May 2003. Jan. 2006 <www.cureparalysisnow.org>.

[104] "Cure Paralysis NOW Advocacy Group." What is an Embryonic Stem Cell (ESC)? Cure Paralysis Now May 2003. Jan. 2006 <www.cureparalysisnow.org>.

[105] One single neural stem cell can divide to make more cells that together form a round hollow structure known as a neurosphere that continues to grow in culture until it is too big. At this point they are disaggregated into single cells. Like cord and embryonic stem cell banks, neural stem cell banks have also been established in various countries and are currently being expanded. "Cure Paralysis NOW Advocacy Group." What is an Embryonic Stem Cell (ESC)? Cure Paralysis Now May 2003. Jan. 2006 <www.cureparalysisnow.org>.

[106] A single pluripotent stem cell has the ability to give rise to types of cells that develop from the three germ layers (mesoderm, endoderm, and ectoderm) from which all the cells of the body arise. The only known sources of human pluripotent stem cells are those isolated and cultured from early human embryos and from fetal tissue originally destined to be part of the gonads. "National Institutes of Health." Stem Cell Information: Executive Summary NIH Aug. 2005. Jul. 2006 <www.stemcells.nih.gov>.

[107] "National Institutes of Health." Stem Cell Information: Executive Summary NIH Aug. 2005. Jul. 2006 <www.stemcells.nih.gov>.

[108] However, scientists such as Dr. Hans Scholer are finding ways to take stem cells from adults and "reprogram" them so they have all the flexibility that an embryonic stem cell has. German Science Weekly Highlight 18. "Reprogramming" is done using human somatic cells (any cell other than egg or sperm) with the aid of special cytoplasmic factors obtained from oocytes so as to dedifferentiate them back into pluripotent stem cells. "National Institutes of Health." Stem Cell Information: Executive Summary NIH Aug. 2005. Jul. 2006 <www.stemcells.nih.gov>.

[109] "National Institutes of Health." Stem Cell Information: Executive Summary NIH Aug. 2005. Jul. 2006 <www.stemcells.nih.gov/info/scireport/execSum.asp>. However, several populations of ASCs have been identified in the brain, particularly in a region known as the hippocampus (which is important for memory). When the cells are removed from the brain of mice and grown in tissue culture, their proliferation and differentiation can be influenced through various growth factors.

[110] "AAAS." Reprogramming Adult Stem Cells News Archives Aug. 2005. Jan. 2006 <www.aaas.org>.

[111] Chad A. Cowan and colleagues merged human embryonic stem cells with human skin cells called fibroblasts, producing hybrid cells that contained both the fibroblast and stem cell chromosomes. The hybrid cells had the appearance, growth rate, and several key genetic characteristics of human embryonic cells, differentiating into cells from each of the three main tissue types that form in a developing embryo. "AAAS." Reprogramming Adult Stem Cells News Archives Aug. 2005. Jan. 2006 <www.aaas.org>. The genesis of the stem cell line should, however, not be forgotten.

[112] "Cure Paralysis NOW Advocacy Group." What is an Embryonic Stem Cell (ESC)? Cure Paralysis Now May 2003. Jan. 2006 <www.cureparalysisnow.org>.

[113] In 2005 University of North Carolina researchers conducted a study of the effects of cord blood transplantation on newborns and infants with Krabbe disease, which is a lethal disease due to the lack of an enzyme (GALC) that breaks down important compounds in the body; the buildup of these substances damages the nerve cells in the central nerve system, destroying many of them and preventing the repair of others. The victim eventually becomes blind, deaf, and unaware of surroundings and fixed in a stiff posture. Average life span is thirteen months. Eleven newborns who had been diagnosed and fourteen older diagnosed infants who were symptomatic all received umbilical cord blood transplantation from unrelated donors who were not perfect matches. All the newborns showed normal neurological development after the transplantation, except for their motor skills. The older infants had minimal neurologic improvement, and their survival rate was no better than that of untreated children. "About." Cord Blood Transplantation Affects Progression of Krabbe Disease Rare/Orphan Diseases 2006. Jan. 2006 <www.rarediseases.about.com/cs/krabbedisease>.

[114] ALD is a degenerative disorder of the fatty white sheath covering nerve fibers known as myelin. Victims are typically male, age 5-10, and have inherited the disease from the x chromosome. Myelin is a complex fatty neural tissue that insulates nerves. Without it, nerves are unable to conduct an impulse, leading to increasing disability. The most severe form of the disease is characterized by a failure to develop, seizures, adrenal insufficiency, and degeneration of visual and auditory function. "Wikipedia." Adrenoleukodystrophy Wikipedia 2006. Aug. 2006 <www.en.wikipedia.org>. ALD is primarily treated through bone marrow or umbilical cord transplant. The goal is to get healthy stem cells to find their way into the brain, express the functioning ALD protein, and prevent or reverse the brain damage. The specifics of this therapy have not been scientifically proven.

However, it is accepted within the ALD community that, if certain patient and donor criteria are met, a favorable outcome may be anticipated; the procedure has an anticipated forty percent mortality rate due to the high doses of chemotherapy necessary to suppress the immune system. "The Stop ALD Foundation." Stem Cell Transplants: An Explanation of Bone Marrow Transplants (BMTs) and Umbilical Cord Blood Transplants (UCBTs) Current Therapies Winter 2004/ 2005. Feb. 2006 <www.stopald.org>.

[115] ALS, like SMA, is characterized by alpha motor neuron degeneration in the anterior horn of the spine. A study published in 2003 found that cord blood transfusion into the systemic circulation of mice delayed the disease progression at least 2-3 weeks and increased the life span of diseased mice. Additionally, transplanted cells survived 10-12 weeks after infusion during which time they entered regions of motor neuron degeneration in the brain and spinal cord. "NCBI Pub/Med." Intravenous Administration of Human Umbilical Cord Blood Cells in a Mouse Model of Amyotrophic Lateral Sclerosis: Distribution, Migration, and Differentiation PubMed abstract Jun. 2003. Feb. 2006 <www.ncbi.nlm.nih.gov>.

[116] "… if you want motor neurons [from USBSCs], forget it." Dr. Douglas Kerr. "… I think there is a strong possibility that nothing would happen." Dr. Kathy Swoboda. FSMA "Families of Spinal Muscular Atrophy." Transcript of Q&A FSMA Research 2005. Jan. 2006 <www.fsma.org>. The primary reasons for the aversion to cord stem cells: (1) the cells are already partially differentiated, (2) no neurons come from them under natural situations, and (3) the high mortality rate of the transplant procedure (twenty percent) from the chemotherapy or radiation that is necessary to down-regulate the possibility of an immune response, thus causing susceptibility to bacteria, viruses and other pathogens. "Families of Spinal Muscular Atrophy." Transcript of Q&A FSMA Research 2005. Jan. 2006 <www.fsma.org>. Both doctors favor embryonic stem cells.

[117] In October of 2000, preimplantation genetic diagnosis (PGD) made headlines when a Colorado couple used assisted reproductive technology to have a baby (named Adam) whose umbilical cord stem cells could cure his six-year-old sister's Fanconi anemia. When Adam was a ball of blastomere cells, researchers at Reproductive Genetics Institute at Illinois Masonic Medical Center separated and probed one of his cells and confirmed that his genome was free of the Fanconi anemia gene and also a match for his sister in terms of leukocyte antigens (unmentioned was how many blastomere's the doctors had tested before Adam).

Researchers implanted the remainder of Adam (a ball of cells) into his mother's uterus, and Adam was born. Physicians infused his umbilical cord stem cells into his sister and she was cured without having an immune response or the need for immunorepression drugs. This bred moral concerns about selective breeding. It also begged the question: what would have happened to Blastomere Adam if he wasn't a match or if he had the genetic defect? Lewis, Ricki. "The Scientist." Pre-implantation Genetic Diagnosis: The Next Big Thing? Research Nov. 2000 Jan. 2006 <www.the-scientist.com>.

[118] The moral issue again would be: what to do if the embryo is not a carrier? It would not matter if it were not an exact match as a somatic cell from the diseased patient could mix with the line. There are other moral concerns than the killing of unused embryos. Are in vitro fertilization and PGD the first steps down a slippery slope to create babies for use as spare parts? Is it ethical to create a "designer baby" in order to treat or cure a sibling? "Science and Theology News." An Alternate Use for PGD Science and Theology News 2006. Jan. 2006 <www.religioustolerance.org>.

[119] The Church and Science are in agreement that life begins at conception, not when it is convenient to recognize it as such. This fact is indisputable. In hESCs procedures, while one embryo is allowed to grow into a baby, another is destroyed for its cells. One argument for embryonic stem cell research is: "They are just going to throw the embryos away anyway." This argument acknowledges that the embryos are life, but that somehow being caught in a bad situation, such as being frozen, justifies or even necessitates experimentation. The argument continues: some good must come out of this. Thus, proponents of embryonic stem cell research blur the issue by using terms and phrases that characterize the embryo as "not a person". (Recall Ron Reagan Jr.'s speech before a recent Democratic National Convention, in which he said that the cells at issue "have no fingers and toes, no brain or spinal cord, no thoughts, no fears." Simply because an embryo is not in the final form of a child, it is no less human. God's plan (in the form of genetic material) is already in place. Every person on earth begins from one cell that predetermines sex, hair color, eye color, length, and other factors. Peterson, Cynthia M. Stem Cell Research." Women for Faith and Family Oct. 2004. Jan. 2006 <www.wff.org>.

[120] The only known sources of human pluripotent stem cells are those isolated and cultured from early human embryos and from fetal tissue that was destined

to be part of the gonads. "National Institutes of Health." Stem Cell Information: Executive Summary NIH Aug. 2005. Jul. 2006 <www.stemcells.nih.gov>.

[121] "Cure Paralysis NOW Advocacy Group." What is an Embryonic Stem Cell (ESC)? Cure Paralysis Now May 2003. Jan. 2006 <www.cureparalysisnow.org>.

[122] Results of this study were presented at the annual meeting of The Society for Neuroscience in New Orleans. The researchers introduced neural stem cells (isolated from human fetal tissue in 1998) into the spinal fluid of mice and rats paralyzed by an animal virus that attacks motor neurons. After eight weeks, noticeable improvement was apparent. The cells migrated to the ventral horn, a region of the spinal cord containing bodies of motor nerve cells. Fifty percent of the stem-cell treated rodents recovered the ability to place the soles of one or both of their hind feet behind them. As a result, Dr. Jeffrey Rothstein claimed: "Under the best research circumstances, stems cells could be used in early clinical trials within two years." "Hopkins Medicine." Stem Cells Graft in Spinal Cord Restore Movement in Paralyzed Mice Hopkins Medicine Nov. 2000. Feb. 2006 <www.hopkinsmedicine.org/press>. See also: "National Institutes of Health." Rebuilding the Nervous System with Stem Cells Stem Cell Information 2006. Jul. 2006 <www.stemcells.nih.gov>.

[123] See <www.fsma.org>. The obvious implication here is that hESCs have the potential cure for all types of paralysis whether due to injury or disease. The motor neurons were produced by using high purity cells (95%) from hESCs. Most derivations of cell populations from hESCs have been less than twenty percent pure.

[124] In newborns, the motor neurons will likely have the ability to grow connections out to the muscles because the distance is short. With older patients, this would prove more difficult, as they are significantly larger. Clinical trials are planned for late 2006 for human subjects of spinal cord injury. The second trial will be for SMA Type I. "FSMA." Stem Cells For the Treatment of SMA Research, Winter 2005/06. Feb. 2006 <www.fsma.org>. Also see: Ackerman, Todd. "Chron.com." Scientists See Value in Both Embryonic, Adult Stem Cells Houston and Texas, Jul. 2006. Jul. 2006. <www.chron.com>.

[125] "Motor Neuron Disease Association." Stem Cells and Motor Neuron Disease June 2005. In an exciting observation that contradicts traditional understanding of ASCs, scientists report that it is possible to convert bone marrow stem cells

into other types of cells, including nerve cells and muscle cells (rather than blood cells only). This observation is not without dispute, however. For example, some scientists contend that converted bone marrow stem cells have a similar structure and shape to nerve cells, but it is not clear whether they can carry electrical messages to and from the right places in the body. It is important to understand however, that neural stem cells generally originate from the brains of nine to fifteen week-old aborted fetuses.

[126] Cromie, William J. "The Harvard University Gazette." Nerve Cell Clones Repair Brain Damage Harvard Gazetter Archives, Jan. 1999. Aug. 2006 <www.hno.harvard.edu/gazette/1999>. "We cloned cells once from a single fetus, then expanded their numbers."

[127] This demonstrates that neural stem cells transplanted into the central nervous system integrate, migrate and differentiate into multiple cell types according their local environment. This could lead to an effective treatment for single-gene neurodegnearive diseases such as SMA. "Children's Hospital Boston." MRRC Project(s) The Snyder Laboratory 2006. Aug. 2006 <www. childrenshospital.org>. See also: Cromie, William J. "The Harvard University Gazette." Nerve Cell Clones Repair Brain Damage Harvard Gazetteer Archives, Jan. 1999. Aug. 2006.

[128] "Special Child." Neural Stem Cell Therapies Information Avenue Archives, Nov. 1999. Aug. 2006 <www.specialchild.com>.

[129] "Motor Neuron Disease Association." Stem Cells and Motor Neuron Disease June 2005. For example, initially researchers thought that stem cells were replacing the existing damaged nerve cells. This is now thought to be unlikely. It is now believed that stem cells may have a more indirect effect. Scientists suggest that stem cells can help damaged motor neurons to survive by providing neurotrophic (nerve nourishing) and protective factors.

[130] One problem in transferring this therapy into humans is the relative lengths of the motor neurons involved. New growth of motor neurons in mice is only a few centimeters. In humans the equivalent nerve growth required is as much as a meter. "Motor Neuron Disease Association." Stem Cells and Motor Neuron Disease June 2005.

[131] Stem cells have the ability to "rescue" cells by reducing inflammation, preventing scarring and releasing growth factors that nourish nearby cells. Dr. Evans

Snyder. Lieberman, Bruce. “SignonSanDiego.” Researchers Are in the Biology 101 Stage of Learning the Potentials for Cures The Promise of Stem Cells Dec. 2004. Jul. 2006 <www.signonsandiego.com>.

132 “MDA Publications.” Renewing Muscles and Nerves: Could Stem Cells be the Ultimate Body Repair Kit? Quest Vol. 7 Apr. 2000. Jan. 2006 <www.mdusa.org>.

133 “MDA Publications.” Renewing Muscles and Nerves: Could Stem Cells be the Ultimate Body Repair Kit? Quest Vol. 7 Apr. 2000. Jan. 2006 <www.mdusa.org>. Dr. Kunkel is also responsible for identifying the defective gene responsible for Duchenne muscular dystrophy.

134 “MDA Publications.” Renewing Muscles and Nerves: Could Stem Cells be the Ultimate Body Repair Kit? Quest Vol. 7 Apr. 2000. Jan. 2006 <www.mdusa.org>. However, the level of dystrophin-positive fibers resulting from these initial transplants was not high enough to restore muscle function in mice.

135 The Hox gene encodes for axonal growth, and another gene may shut off the Nogo gene that restricts growth.

136 “National Institutes of Health.” Use of Genetically Modified Stem Cells in Experimental Gene Therapies Stem Cell Information, 2006. Jul. 2006 <www.stemcells.nih.gov>. They can select and work only with those cells that contain both the transgene and produce the therapeutic agent in sufficient quantity.

137 Cells can be programmed to steadily churn out a given amount of therapeutic product. In some cases, it is desirable to program the cells to make large amounts of the therapeutic gene so that the chances that sufficient quantities are secreted and reach the diseased tissue in the patient are high. In other cases, it may be desirable to program the cells to produce the therapeutic gene in a regulated fashion so that the transgene would be active only in response to certain signals, such as drugs administered to the patient to turn the therapeutic transgene on and off. “National Institutes of Health.” Use of Genetically Modified Stem Cells in Experimental Gene Therapies Stem Cell Information, 2006. Jul. 2006 <www.stemcells.nih.gov>.

[138] Thus, myoblasts may not only be useful for treating muscle disorders, such as muscular dystrophy, but also non-muscle disorders such as neurodegenerative diseases. "National Institutes of Health." Use of Genetically Modified Stem Cells in Experimental Gene Therapies Stem Cell Information, 2006. Jul. 2006 <www.stemcells.nih.gov>.

[139] Investigators injected myoblasts containing the transgene for a human nerve growth factor into the muscles of the ALS mice before the onset of the disease symptoms and motor neuron degeneration. The transgene remained active in the muscle for up to twelve weeks. More importantly, the gene therapy successfully delayed the onset of disease symptoms, slowed muscle atrophy, and delayed deterioration of motor skills. "National Institutes of Health." Use of Genetically Modified Stem Cells in Experimental Gene Therapies Stem Cell Information, 2006. Jul. 2006 <www.stemcells.nih.gov>.

[140] However, scientists recently cured melanoma cancer in two patients using gene therapy. Doctors drew blood from the melanoma cancer patients and isolated the white blood cells. New genes were inserted into the cells that created T-receptors that can recognize and destroy the cancer once they are re-injected into the body. Seventeen patients were treated this way; two treatments were successful, and cancer was entirely eliminated from their bodies. Associated Press. "Closer to a Cure." Cape Cod Times 1 Sept. 2006: 2. Of the stem cell-based gene therapy trials that have had a therapeutic goal, approximately one-third have focused upon cancers, one-third on AIDS, and one-third on so-called single-gene therapies. None of these clinical trials is focusing specifically on SMA.

[142] New techniques are being developed that can create embryonic stem cells without harming the embryo. In the August 23, 2006 issue of the journal *Nature* a paper submitted by lead researcher Rober Lanza (of Advanced Cell Technology (ACT), Worcester, Massachusetts) detailed how a single cell plucked from an early human embryo can be coaxed to divide repeatedly in a laboratory dish and grow into a colony of stem cells. Weiss, Rick. "Stem Cell Advance Reported" 23 Aug 2006: 1.

[143] "National Institutes of Health." Use of Genetically Modified Stem Cells in Experimental Gene Therapies Stem Cell Information, 2006. Jul. 2006 <www.stemcells.nih.gov>. Retroviruses are able to do this, and for this reason they are often used as the vehicle for infecting the stem cell and introducing the therapeutic transgene into the chromosomal DNA. However, because hemato-

poietic stem cells are quiescent (meaning that they seldom divide), the therapeutic transgene has usually been too low in amount to attain therapeutic effect. One way of overcoming this problem is to stimulate the hematopoietic stem cells to divide so that the viral vehicles can infect them and insert the therapeutic transgene. However, this manipulation can change other important properties of the hematopoietic stem cells, such a plasticity, self-renewal, and the ability to survive and grow when introduced to the patient.

[144] An autoimmune disease is a condition that results from the formation of antibodies that attack the cells own tissues of an individual's own body. All immune and blood cells develop from multi-potent hematopoietic stem cells that originate in the bone marrow. Upon their departure from the bone marrow, immature T-cells undergo a final maturation process in the thymus, a small organ in the upper chest, before being dispersed to the body with the rest of the immune cells (B cells). Within the thymus, T-cells are "educated" to distinguish between self (the proteins of the body) and nonself (the invading organism's antigens or proteins that induce the formation of an antibody). Within the thymus, the T-cells are selected for their ability to bind to the particular proteins expressed in the individual's body. Collectively, these T-cells are capable of recognizing an almost unlimited number of antigens. However, many immature T-cells have the potential to react with the body's own proteins. To avoid this potential disaster, the thymus provides an environment where T-cells that recognize self-antigens (autoreactive T-cells) are deleted (through apoptosis) or inactivated in a process called tolerance induction. Tolerance usually ensures that T-cells do not attack the self-proteins of the body. Autoimmune diseases arise when this intricate system for the induction and maintenance of immune tolerance fails. The result is the destruction of tissue, such as joints in rheumatoid arthritis, or insulin-producing beta cells of the pancreas in type 1 diabetes, or damage to the kidneys in lupus. "National Institutes of Health." Autoimmune Diseases and the Promise of Stem Cell-Based Therapies Stem Cell Information, 2006. Jul. 2006 <www.stemcells.nih.gov>.

[145] Muscular dystrophy is a family of genetically inherited diseases that attack the muscles. Many of the afflictions are due to a lack of the protein dystrophin that the muscles need as a scaffolding" upon which to build. SMA does not fit into this class for three reasons: (1) the muscles are not afflicted (they merely atrophy due to a lack of use); (2) a lack of dystrophin is not part of SMA; and (3) SMA is attacked from the motor neurons due to a lack of SMN protein (perhaps most

needed in the axons). "Cell Transplants International LLC." Frequently Asked Questions celltherapy.com 2002. Aug. 2006 <www.celltherapy.com>.

[146] "National Institute of Health." Gene Therapy and Stem Cell Approaches for Treatment of Autoimmune diseases NIH 2006. Jul. 2006 <www.stemcells.nih.gov>. One strategy is to block the actions of an inflammatory cytokine (secreted by activated immune cells and inflamed tissues) and to produce long-lasting expression of the intended protein at levels that can be tightly controlled by transferring a gene into cells that encode a "decoy" receptor for that cytokine. For example, in a lupus mouse model, gene transfer of the decoy receptor via DNA injection arrested disease progression. This strategy also prevented onset of diabetes in mice. Another strategy would be to transfer a gene that encodes an anti-inflammatory cytokine, redirecting the auto-inflammatory immune response to a more "tolerant" state. Animal studies have shown promising results by using these approaches. However, similar challenges exist as in other fields of stem cell-gene therapy. For example, one such challenge would be to reliably transfer genetic material into adult and slowly dividing stem cells (including hematopoietic stem cells) and to produce long-lasting expression of the intended protein at levels that can be tightly controlled in response to disease activity.

[147] This may be due to activation of the cysteine protease caspase 3 that appears to be a key event in the execution of apoptosis in the central nervous system. Robertson, George, S. "Blackwell Synergy." Neuroprotection by the Inhibition of Apoptosis Brain Pathology abstract Apr. 2000. Jul. 2006 <www.blackwell-synergy.com>.

[148] Roberson, George, S. "Blackwell Synergy." Neuroprotection by the Inhibition of Apoptosis Brain Pathology abstract Apr. 2000. Jul. 2006 <www.blackwell-synergy.com>. Capase 3 activation has recently been observed in stroke, spinal cord trauma, head injury and Alzheimers' disease patients.

[149] Splicing is an extraordinary process where large chunks of useless and meaningless sequence have accumulated in the genes of all higher organisms. The information is broken up into islands called exons. In order to function, genes need to be processed into RNA. This occurs when a mechanism is created in which a complementary copy of a gene is made, followed by removal of the meaningless sequences. The precious exons are then stitched together. "Univ. Of Leicester biochemistry Dept." Oligos 2006. Jan. 2006 <www.le.ac.u>.

[150] Oligonucleotides (oligos) are short sequences of nucleotides (RNA or DNA) that are often used to amplify almost any piece of DNA because of its binding attributes. Antisense oligos are single strands of DNA or RNA that prevent translation of RNA strands by binding to it. "Wikipedia." Oligonucleotide Wikipedia 2006. Aug. 2006. <www.en.wikipedia.org>.

[151] A leading company in the production of oligos is Illumina. Ilumina's design begins by attaching hundreds of thousands of oligos to glass beads so tiny that several dozen would fit onto the period at the end of this sentence. Brown, Stuart F. "Mindfully." Building DNA Chips Using Tricks from Nanotech and Bioinformatics Soul of New Gene Machines, May 2005. Jul. 2006 <www.mindfully.org>.

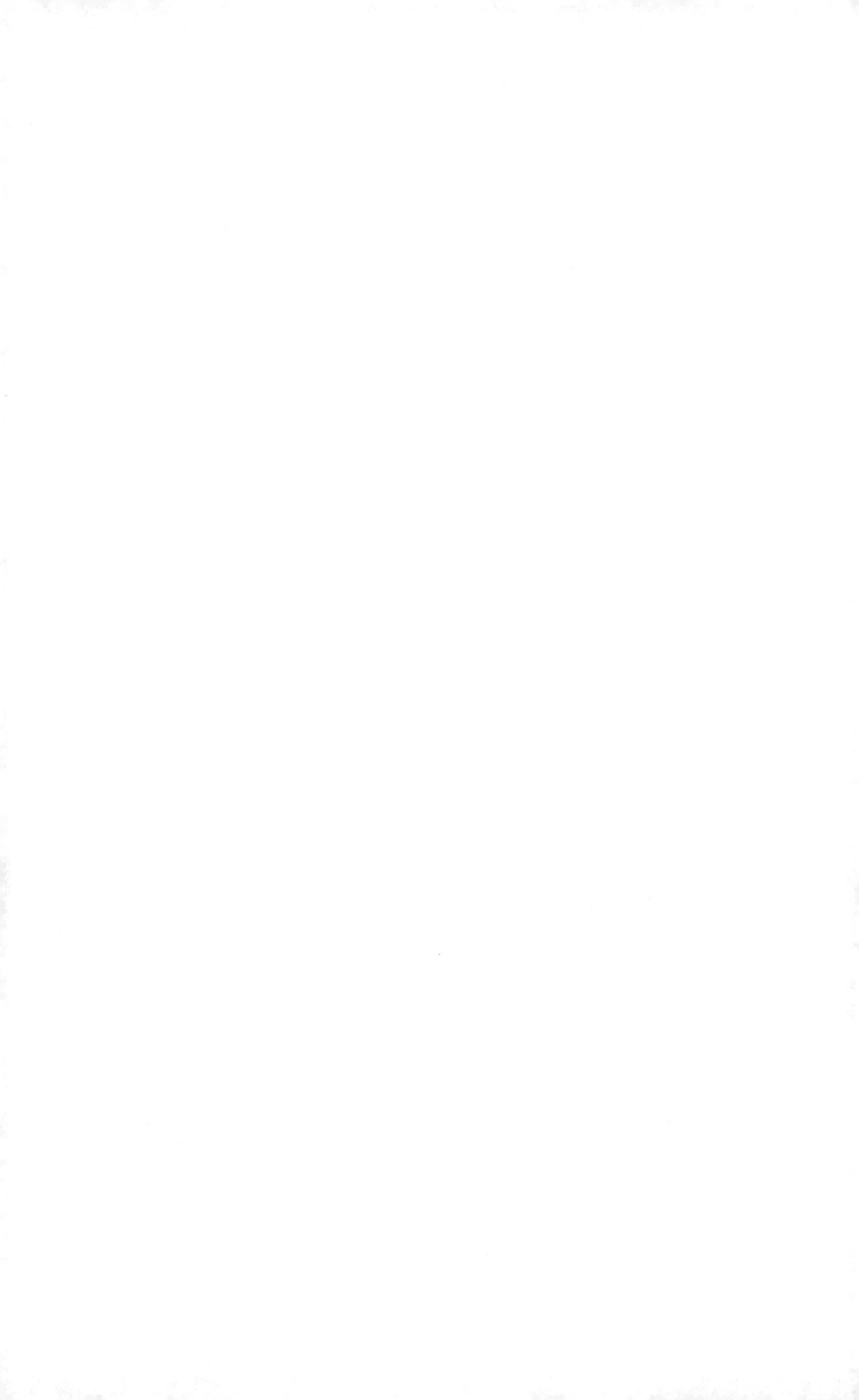

978-0-595-42833-5
0-595-42833-9

www.ingramcontent.com/pod-product-compliance
Lightning Source LLC
Chambersburg PA
CBHW030915180526
45163CB00004B/1837